Intermittent Fasting For Weight Loss

Special Edition - Three Books

*Combine Three Powerful Strategies
For Rapid Fat Loss, Increased Health and
Anti-Aging Benefits*

Michael D Kaiser, Dana Lee

inattention, use, or misuse of the information in question by the reader will render any resulting actions solely under their purview. There are no scenarios in which the publisher or the original author of this work can be in any fashion deemed liable for any hardship or damages that may befall them after undertaking information described herein.

Additionally, the information in the following pages is intended only for informational purposes and should thus be thought of as universal. As befitting its nature, it is presented without assurance regarding its prolonged validity or interim quality. Trademarks that are mentioned are done without written consent and can in no way be considered an endorsement from the trademark holder. No medical advice is being given in the book.

Book One

Intermittent Fasting

Burn Fat, Lose Weight, Become Energetic and Happy

Use The Power Of Your Body To Lose Weight and Increase Health

Michael D Kaiser

Table of Contents

Introduction

The world of dieting is growing increasingly chaotic. People are confused as to what "diet" will work and what foods are safe to eat, even healthy foods. This has led to the creation of prehistoric diets that are trying to model what a caveman or pre-historic man/woman ate, as that should be the most optimal diet for humans today. Although it works for many people, we are not cave people anymore nor are we spending 15 hours a day hunting and gathering food just to survive.

The other problem facing so many people today is that we have so much rich food available to us everywhere we go, it constantly surrounds us and is easily available. Most of the food is processed or infused with chemicals that cause it to not be digested properly which drains our energy during the day, making it difficult to focus or work.

I personally simply use a mostly vegetarian whole foods diet in my daily intermittent fasting, even though I have tried many other diets and foods, I found that the whole foods works best for me, in intermittent fasting, which includes 2-3 weekly servings of healthy fish, chicken or beef. It wasn't until I started intermittent fasting that I saw amazing results. At first I thought it was my diet or maybe the sprints I was doing, or the supplement I was taking, but no, it was fasting for 15-16 hours a day that was making the changes.

The biggest change was the reduction of what little sub-cutaneous fat I still had, so that my abs were finally visible, and my veins became visible too. Then the biomarkers in my blood increased, and when I became very strict about eating only whole natural foods with no added oils, sugar or other chemicals that disrupt the body, things really became amazing. Today I often get comments that I appear to be in my early thirties or even late twenties, and I am 41 years old as of this writing. I attribute a lot of the health benefits to INTERMITTENT FASTING, but for optimal health it is really going to be many factors (food choices, exercise, attitude, sun exposure, genetics, etc.)

This book is a basic introductory to Intermittent Fasting for the beginner

It will get you started with the following basics:

- What Intermittent Fasting is and how it works.
- What popular Intermittent Fasting diets are on the market now.
- How to customize one that works for you and your lifestyle.
- How to integrate it into your life so that it becomes a habit and not a "diet"

The first step will not always be the easiest, which is why the information you will find in the following chapters is so important to take to heart, as they are concepts that can be put into action immediately.

I personally started my own intermittent fasting program in 2015 and it was what ended my plateau I found myself in. I was already very athletic and trying to eat healthy. I permanently lost an additional 12 pounds of fat from intermittent fasting for only a few months. I was already in great shape, ran, jogged, sprinted and cycled almost daily. The biggest discovery I made from intermittent fasting is that I get full really fast when I do eat, so I really do not eat that much. You will probably discover the same effect. More importantly, the biggest benefit I received for fasting daily is the health benefits I feel, the less I ate all the time, the better I felt. It was very strange, but I realized that when I WASN'T eating, I felt great. That's when I discovered that eating through-out the day is not for me anymore, and is more of a strain than anything else.

The following chapters will discuss the preparedness you will need to really lose weight and gain the health benefits of intermittent fasting. This means that you will want to consider the quality of your food, including the potential issues raised by their quality, how they can best be utilized in a meal, as well as various tools you might need to keep your mind focused on the task at hand.

<u>Chapter One</u>

The History of Fasting

The intermittent fasting diet, invented by Ori Hofmekler, is based on a daily food cycle that includes two phases: underfeeding during the day and overfeeding during the evening-night.

The phase of underfeeding should last all day, applying the rules of the intermittent fasting diet. This naturally stimulates the sympathetic nervous system (SNS) which promotes vigilance, competitiveness, and energy expenditure. During this time, the body moves into a negative energy balance and is therefore forced to burn stored fat to produce energy.

During the underfeeding phase, the consumption of food consisting mostly of raw fruits and vegetables, soups, and small amounts of protein foods should be minimized.

The major food intake phase takes place during the evening-night hours.

This is the moment when the main meal should be consumed when you can eat as much as you want from all the food groups but still following certain dietary patterns, which we will dwell on more later.

Physically active individuals may require more energy and special types of fuel (fats or carbohydrates), depending on the nature and level of their physical activity. The phase of food abundance causes the activation of the parasympathetic nervous system (SNP), which promotes relaxation and recovery.

During this phase, the body moves towards a positive energy balance while creating a general anabolic-constructive state. This is the moment when the body recovers, builds the tissues and fills the energy reserves.

An example of Intermittent fasting were the soldiers of the Roman Empire who were subjected to major stresses for wars and large displacements. They were trained to fight and possessed powerful bodies and important muscle masses, so they carried a lot of energy accumulated in the periods of rest.

More specifically, the Hofmekler model, which also partly refers to intermittent fasting and caloric restriction studies, provides only one large meal a day after 10-12 hours of fasting or limited to the intake of small protein snacks or fruit or vegetable juices.

Under these conditions, the organism would interpret the fast as a sort of state of emergency and consequently synthesize a whole series of hormones that favor the transformation of fats into energy (growth hormone, adrenaline, noradrenaline) and improve the physical response to the environmental circumstances.

According to Hofmekler, the fact that breakfast is considered the most important meal of the day has no scientific basis, while the human body would be more alert and efficient if you keep fasting until evening.

Man is, by nature, a nocturnal eater programmed to work and fast during the day and eat and rest during the night, while it would be customary to consume his meals during the day which, going against nature, promotes the development of obesity, diabetes, heart attack and stroke.

During the day, you will have to eat completely natural foods, such as vegetables, a little fruit, and small amounts of protein.

The goal of the intermittent fasting diet is to create a lifestyle that imitates that of our predecessors from prehistory to ancient Rome (primitives and gladiators).

To summarize everything, we could say that this food model is based on the assumption that nourishing the body by supporting the circadian rhythms of primitive man is functional to the maintenance of physical form and health, as it enhances the use of nutrients and the transformation of body fat into energy while at the same time increasing resistance to stress.

The author has "engraved" the real commandments that "the warrior" subjected to this diet will have to follow. Those are:

- Provide your body with all the essential nutrients (vitamins, minerals, EFA, amino acids, and probiotics). Introduce all the aromas, flavors, textures and colors possible.

- When possible, cyclically rotate the days when carbohydrates, proteins, or fats dominate the caloric percentages taken.

- Avoid foods containing hormones, pesticides, chemical additives, sugar alcohols, artificial sweeteners, and excess fructose.

- Do not eat foods that contain high-glycemic carbohydrates on their own.

- Exercise regularly even during the underfeeding phase.

Avoid wrong food combinations such as:

- Wheat and sugar
- Starch and fats
- Walnuts and parmesan
- Carbohydrates and alcohol

The body is designed to eat this way.

The cyclicity between negative energetic and positive energy balance of genes known as "parsimonious genes" improves human survival chances. This is measured by the ability to improve energy use, performance, and health. Intermittent fasting lets you turn on biological switches that improve human survival day by day.

In the morning, just wake up, and on an empty stomach, we have 3 main substances in circulation:

- testosterone – every man has a peak of it in the morning;
- cortisol – a stress hormone, extremely lipolytic hormone;
- catecholamines — adrenaline and noradrenaline, pure energy.

All these hormones increase energy aggression and mental clarity, and they are stimulated by the empty stomach.

In this fasting phase, you will lose weight and water.

If you start eating at this stage of the day, you would raise insulin and GH—hormones that make you calm, relaxed but little aggressive, lazy, feel weak, and immediately store the energies and lower the 3 hormones above.

The blood then moves away from the muscles to go to the stomach for digestion and therefore less blood to the muscles.

Another positive outcome from fasting is its purification effect on the liver and the kidney.

In the overeating phase, you have to start eating less tasty foods and then move on to tastier foods, so you will start with the intake of salad, vegetables, proteins—then finish with the richest carbohydrate foods.

It will be important to introduce a wide variety of foods—both from the point of view of flavor, consistency and color—to get all the nutritive principles (macro and micronutrients).

Chapter Two

What is Wrong With Our Modern Diets?

Have you ever wondered why we eat? It is one of those simple questions behind our discovery of the complex mechanisms that run our lives. The first reason why we eat is that it allows us to grow from being an infant until we reach our maturity as an adult. The second function of nutrition is to conserve life. Food gives energy to our body and maintains a caloric level sufficient to conserve the temperature of the body of each species. In this case, human beings have a normal body temperature of 37 degrees Celsius.

What happens if food is not consumed? The body takes calories from the fat tissue, which is temporarily stored mostly in your belly when you eat. A good health refers to keeping the process of food input and food expenditure in balance. If you eat too much, you go beyond the natural purpose for which fat deposits exist. This will make you obese.

In the richest countries, obesity is an increasingly widespread phenomenon. Various explanations are given as to why there is a widespread obesity in such countries. For some, the impulse to eat beyond measure comes from an ancestral hunger, sort of a command left in the brain and ready to be activated in the presence of food.

For others, the explanation is psychological. In fact, we create an abnormal situation with this almost neurotic need for excessive nutrition. Just look at how many mothers overfeed their children today.

Positive food education

Today, everything is turned upside down, and it is often the children who blackmail their parents by threatening not to eat if they do not turn up the television or condescend to their desires. Instead, the golden rule is to eat little. Not only because of the cardiovascular risks related to being overweight, but also because more food is introduced, and more risks are incurred for cancer. The risk of cancer is proportional to the amount of food that is introduced: more food, more risks. This is why I decided to write this book: to make an invitation to frugality and, maybe, to inspire parents to be stricter with their children.

Many food pathologies are linked to a culture that has lost sight of what really is necessary to survive. Diseases such as anorexia and bulimia did not exist almost 30-40 years ago when there was education in food and attention to its good use. As Bismarck said, you can forget the rules of healthy eating on your birthday, but you do not have to celebrate your birthday every day.

Even this apparently simple question proposes to our attention the mechanism of life on Earth and its conservation and propagation. It is a complex alchemy, which occurs in a regime of mutual exchange between those that our elementary school books defined, with a suggestive word, the "kingdoms of nature—" mineral, vegetable, and animal. The plant world absorbs carbon dioxide from the atmosphere and transforms it into plants, which, in turn, produce oxygen.

The animal world behaves in an opposite way and is the protagonist of a reverse project: it absorbs oxygen and burns it, producing carbon dioxide. The Earth lives on this harmonious relationship: on the one hand, plants produce what animals consume, and the product of this process serves the vegetable world to live.

And now, let's go back to the history of man. Man is a primate, which means that he is a modified monkey, and the monkey has maintained very basic metabolic characteristics. Primates have been and still are vegetarians and also interact with the plant world because they basically eat fruit.

The flowers, from which the fruit will then be born, are colored and fragrant because they have to attract pollinating insects that allow fertilization. The fruits, equally colored and fragrant, attract animals, including humans. However, this harmony and this synergy between different kingdoms and worlds at some point in human history started to suffer from a great problem: the great glaciations. The plants disappeared almost completely. Many vegetarian animals perished miserably.

The human species was saved, and from a vegetarian species became a carnivore one. The turning point of human nutrition was the ice that covered the planet. Men became carnivorous, but also maintained the metabolism of a vegetarian primate. In short, our organism is programmed for the consumption of fruit and vegetables, and to return largely to this type of food can only benefit us.

We should follow the example of our ancestors' peasants.

Mediterranean Diet

The so-called Mediterranean diet—based on vegetables, fruit, and pasta—has been proven effective in preventing diseases such as cardiovascular diseases, obesity, diabetes and cancer.

The return to a Mediterranean diet has contributed, together with more effective drugs, to the reduction of mortality from cardiovascular diseases. The Mediterranean diet is the diet that has handed down to us the peasant population of America and of all those countries that overlook the Mediterranean Sea. You ate a little meat, a lot of fish (if you lived on the shores of the sea), cereals, pasta, legumes, vegetables, and fruits. It was a poor but balanced diet, and it was enough to sustain life.

The situation today is a tragic paradox; on one side, there is the poor world starving; on the other, the rich world dying of obesity.

What is intermittent fasting?

Although it may seem absurd, fasting is good for the mind and the body. There are many forms of "the fasting diet," but the type that has been rediscovered in recent times is that of intermittent fasting.

The diet varies: from allowing the consumption of calories only for a certain period of the day (usually from six to twelve hours) to drastic caloric reduction for 48 hours—until complete fasting every week.

The studies on intermittent fasting are innumerable, many of which are still "work in progress," but significant benefits are being highlighted on several aspects.

In addition to losing weight, intermittent fasting would also improve blood pressure and help the body dispose of fat by going into ketosis.

Positive indicators also seem to be related to the reduction of cancer risk, especially breast cancer—yet they are still in progress.

Returning to weight, it has been proven that the more the body accuses the fast, the more it uses fat as fuel, thus entering into ketosis.

Not only that: there would be a positive feedback as well regarding a significant reinforcement of neural connections with consequent improvement of memory and mood.

Those who practice intermittent fasting report feeling more lucid and focused during fasting.

Scientists would argue that ketogenic diets would help to fight diseases like Alzheimer's - precisely because of this cognitive improvement at the hands of fasting, which also improves mood.

Intermittent fasting would seem to be propaedeutic even for diabetes.

A fast that includes, for example, a few days without particular restrictions on food—always following a healthy and controlled diet—followed by a very narrow diet of 5 days, would bring significant improvements to those with high blood sugar.

Prof. Valter Longo is considered the guru of food and anti-aging, and his studies on human aging have led him to develop the Diet Mima Fasting (another type of fasting diet).

DMF is able to give the healthy and anti-aging benefits of fasting while at the same time eating normally the remaining twenty-five days a month.

It is not certain that intermittent fasting can bring about the same benefits, even if it is possible. Professor Longo's recommendation is not to abuse the term "intermittent fasting." It is known that some forms of fasting—how to consistently restrict food during one or two days a week or eat only at certain times—bring health benefits, but it is not yet known whether this applies to all types of fasting.

Chapter Three

The Science of How it Works

Before getting into the details of intermittent fasting, I'd like to spend some time talking about the basics of nutrition. When we talk about diet and nutrition, we often do not know the principles that underlie our very existence and, above all, our physical well-being. We limit ourselves to eating something that others have advised us, and we often take pills and tablets advertised, which not only have no use but wrapped up can even be harmful to our health and our finances.

In order not to get lost in the sea of nutrition, the first useful thing is to make an overview of food principles and daily human needs.

Let's start by saying that all foods can be classified into five large food groups:
- carbohydrates
- proteins (or protides)
- fats (or lipids)
- vitamins
- minerals

Carbohydrates are the elements most present in our diet. They are made up of two main elements—carbon and water—that when joined together give rise to the simplest of sugars, glucose. Aggregating then into larger molecules, they form two different groups of carbohydrates: simple sugars (consisting of a few molecules of glucose) and complex sugars (formed by long chains of glucose). A subsequent classification is that which divides them into monosaccharides (a sugar molecule), disaccharides (two molecules), and polysaccharides (more than two molecules).

There are about 200 different types of carbohydrates, and oftentimes, they take the name from the food in which they are in large quantities. For instance, there are some carbohydrates called fructose, lactose, maltose, but also sucrose and starch. Carbohydrates are mainly from vegetables, and their function is purely energetic and makes up the basis of human nutrition—providing about 4 calories per gram/weight. They are found in large quantities in pasta, rice, potatoes, fruit, bread, flour as well as in legumes.

The cells of our body transform all the carbohydrates introduced into the simplest form, glycogen, which, once oxidized into the cellular mitochondria, provides energy for rapid and above-all clean use, i.e. without waste. These must, therefore, represent the basis of our nutrition and must provide about 60-65% of the energy needs.

However, it is rare to have to carry out a glucosidic supplementation. In fact, they are so widely present in all foods, that perhaps we should think about reducing their consumption.

Fats, on the other hand, are complex acidic structures found in both animal and vegetable foods. Like carbohydrates, fats also have a purely energetic function, with a different caloric value. Lipids bring about 9 calories per gram/weight, and their burning rate is very slow. In fact, before being used, fats must be transformed into simpler elements, which the cell can then oxidize to obtain energy. In their complex form, on the other hand, they are easily stored as fat storage, which is the energy reserve of our body. Fats are often divided into saturated and unsaturated, depending on the type of chemical bond that forms the molecule. To simplify, we can say that saturated fats are "bad" **and harmful to our arteries**—these include cholesterol, glycerol, hydrogenated fats, fats contained in butter and margarine, palm oil, and most fats of animal origin.

The "good" fats instead are the unsaturated fats or those contained in nuts, avocados and fish fats (omega 3 and omega 6), and lecithin (abundant in soybeans).

In addition to energy capacity, fats are involved in many organic activities, including hormone synthesis and cell membrane construction. Their function is therefore vital, and our energy needs should be covered by lipids in the measure of 15-20%.

The integration of fats is very rare, as we usually tend to consume more than we should since they are the vehicle of taste and make us better appreciate the foods we ingest.

When it comes to proteins, it is a totally different story. They are composed of complex chains of amino acids joined together by peptide bonds. These amino acids can bind together in number, proportions, and different forms—giving rise to an almost infinite series of specific proteins.

There are 21 amino acids, 8 of which are called "essential," because our body is not able to synthesize them. In fact, human RNA possesses protein synthesis codes for only 13 amino acids and is able to process proteins that contain only these elements. For a complete protein range, it is necessary to take the remaining 8 amino acids, called essential amino acids, from the outside through eating.

Animal and vegetable proteins are made of the same amino acids—with a substantial difference. While each animal protein contains all 21 amino acids (in different proportions, depending on the protein itself), in the proteins coming from vegetables, there is always something missing. Some plant foods, therefore, contain certain amino acids but do not contain others. It becomes important, then, in the case of a vegetarian diet, to know how to combine the various products so that all the necessary elements are introduced. As we said, this does not apply to animal proteins, which are called "noble" because they are complete.

From an energetic point of view, protides are similar to carbohydrates, bringing about 4 calories per gram/weight. Unfortunately, the energy obtained from proteins is not as clean, because as a result of oxidation at the cellular level, nitrogen is released, which then evolves into free radicals, accelerating the cellular aging process.

The energetic process of proteins is just a *fallback* of the body in the event of an actual need for calories. Normally, protides are used for "plastic" purposes, i.e. they are used in the construction, repair, and renewal of all body structures—such as muscles, bones, cells, organs, apparatuses, and tissues, in general. It can be said that the human body is composed of 70% water, and the rest of it is proteins. To maintain itself, the human body, therefore, needs a certain daily protein intake, which should be about one gram per kilogram of body weight (a man of 80 kilograms should take 80 grams of protein per day). However, this proportion can range between 0.70 grams per kilogram/weight (the minimum to remain healthy) up to a maximum of 1.5 grams per kilogram/weight. Beyond this threshold, you risk that the proteins are used for energetic purposes would rise to many free radicals and other problems related to kidneys and liver. Ultimately, the daily heat intake of proteins should be 15-20%.

The integration of proteins may be necessary in the case of a vegetarian diet, while it's not recommended in a varied diet, including animal foods. Moreover, the assimilation of protides for plastic use is about 4 grams per hour, so we can assume that the body has more means of using them for energy. However, the proteins taken through supplements are less similar than those taken through normal nutrition, as they are metabolized with a certain amount of carbohydrates and vitamins (especially B12).

Another important part of nutrition is the macro group of vitamins. They are organic compounds essential to life and development that normally the human body cannot synthesize and must, therefore, take with food. They are found in large quantities in vegetables and fruits. Many vitamins are sensitive to high temperatures, so it is advisable to take these foods raw. Moreover, some of them deteriorate over time, becoming bioavailable—this is why it is preferable to eat freshly picked fruits and vegetables.

Each vitamin has a specific function, which can vary from the metabolic one (e.g. B12) to the protective one of the blood vessels (vitamin C). The deficiency of a certain vitamin, usually called avitaminosis, can cause specific diseases, such as scurvy in the case of vitamin C deficiency.

Vitamins are distinguished between two categories: water-soluble ones (which means they can be melted in water) and liposoluble ones (melted in fats). Our body is able to store the fat-soluble vitamins (A, D, E, K, and F), while it cannot retain the water-soluble vitamins (C, B1, B2, B5, B6, B12, H, PP) that are easily eliminated in the urine. The latter, in fact, should be taken several times throughout the day. It is also worthy to note that fat-soluble vitamins, which are stored in body fat, have a slower process of elimination. This can cause, in the case of a high intake, a state of toxicity, thus creating very serious dysfunctions. Therefore, if an integration of water-soluble vitamins can be made lightly, we must instead pay maximum attention when it comes to the fat-soluble ones, which should be integrated only in case of established deficiency.

The last food group is one of the minerals and inorganic elements (i.e. without biological carbon) that cover multiple functions. They are often called mineral salts, but this is an improper name since most minerals are devoid of the salt part. Rather, they are single elements present in nature—metals and non-metals—which use water as a vehicle to pass from the earth to the plants and therefore to the animals that feed on them.

They are divided into three groups: macro-elements, micro-elements, and oligo-elements. This division is established on the basis of the daily requirement of the elements, which can vary from 100 milligrams/day for the macro-elements (calcium, phosphorus, potassium, etc.), to less than 200 micrograms/day for the oligo-elements (manganese, chromium, cobalt, etc.).

Although their presence in the body is around 5%/6% of the body weight, they are of vital importance, as they participate in many cellular and metabolic functions. Just think, for instance, about iron, which plays an important part in the cardiovascular system; or calcium, which is a fundamental element of bones and teeth. They must, therefore, be eaten on a regular basis, as the body expels them through the excretory apparatus through urine, feces, and sweat. A varied diet in which vegetables, fruit, meat, fish, eggs, and dried fruit are added, provides the optimal amount of all the necessary minerals.

Mineral deficiency, just like vitamins, can lead to specific diseases, such as iron deficiency anemia, or it can even aggravate diseases such as osteoporosis in the case of calcium deficiency. A certain quantity of minerals is therefore vital, but their excess can instead lead to real phenomena of poisoning. Hence, it would be good to stay away from the saline and mineral supplements, unless there's an ascertained shortage. Most importantly, before starting the intake through supplements, it is advisable to seek medical advice.

Chapter Four

Keys to Success

Tips and Tricks with Intermittent Fasting

The idea of starting a diet can be daunting, especially if you are not mentally prepared to face such a change. When the mind is calm and prepared, sticking to a healthy food program is much simpler. With the right preparation, you will be able to effectively achieve your goals, and you will make it less difficult not to fall into temptation during the journey.

Be aware of the recurring negative thoughts related to food.

Oftentimes, our diets fail because of our beliefs related to food and eating. Try to become aware of your food beliefs and make an effort to change your mentality.

We often think that on special occasions, it is ok to let go a bit. There's nothing wrong with eating a little more from time to time, but be honest with yourself about what you consider "special occasions." When events like eating away from home, business lunches, office parties, and other small events all become excuses to let yourself binge, the failure of the diet is just around the corner. Try, therefore, to re-evaluate what occasions can be considered as "special" and when it is better to stick to your original diet plan.

Do you use food as a reward?

Many think that after a long busy day, it is normal to deserve to go out for dinner or eat an entire tub of ice cream. Look for alternative ways to reward yourself, which do not include food. For example, take a long hot bath, buy a new dress, or go to the cinema. There are many ways to reward yourself without using food.

The importance of listening to your body

Dissociate food from certain activities.

Food is closely linked to numerous rituals. Giving up sugar and fat may not be easy when we emotionally associate them with certain habits. Make a conscious effort to break these dangerous associations.

Try to be aware of the times you eat too much or make bad food choices, both in terms of food and the things you drink. Whenever you go to the cinema, do you buy Coca-Cola and popcorn? Cannot say "no" to a few glasses of wine during the evenings out? Cannot imagine a Saturday morning without coffee and donuts? If so, take the extra mile to commit to chopping these associations.

Try changing associations by replacing harmful foods with healthier ones. For example, when you spend the evening out, dedicate it to a board game instead of focusing on drinking. On Saturday mornings, have breakfast with coffee, yogurt, and fresh fruits. If, at the end of the day, you tend to try to relax through eating, replace the food with a good book or some music.

It is not just about calories.

In the end, you will be more likely to be able to stick to your diet by committing yourself to change your negative behaviors rather than just keeping your calories under control. Try to become aware of when you eat and why you do it. Even if it is only half a biscuit, ask yourself if you are allowing it because you think you have had a bad day. Do you tend to eat because you are hungry or because you feel bored? If you do it out of boredom, try to get rid of this bad habit. Even if you do not exceed the calories, always try to use common sense. Do not eat the wrong foods for the wrong reasons.

Ask for help.

Changing is not easy, and sometimes, we are not able to do it on our own. Ask for help from friends and family. Let them know you are trying to lose weight, and pray to support yourself. Make sure they know they do not have to invite you to parties where cheap food and alcohol will be served. In addition, ask to be able to vent with them in moments when you will feel particularly frustrated or tempted. Share your goals with all the people living under your own roof.

Establish contained and realistic goals.

Many people tend to sabotage their diet by placing the bar of expectations too high. If you want to be able to stick to your plans, set goals achievable.

Remember that a balanced diet allows you to lose about ½-1 kilo a week, no more. If you intend to lose weight faster than that, prepare to fail.

Initially, you should have cautious goals, so you will be more likely to be able to reach them and have the motivation to continue. Unspecific intentions, such as "This week, I will eat vegetables every day," and something like, "The next time I eat out of the house, I will order a salad instead of potato chips," are valid starting points that can lead you to the road to success.

Keep a diary.

If you want your diet to be successful, you cannot exempt yourself from being responsible. Go out and buy a diary that will accompany you along the entire route. Record everything you eat every day, and keep a calorie count. A tangible account will force you to notice your bad habits and motivate you to develop new ones.

Plan your meals.

Planning meals and snacks in advance will help you not to give in to temptations. In the days before the start of the diet, make a list of healthy recipes that you intend to prepare. Try to get ahead, for example, by buying or cutting the necessary ingredients. If you want, you can also cook soups and vegetables to keep in the refrigerator—they will be very useful for the first week lunches.

Focus on concrete behavior.

Limiting yourself to making analyses in abstract terms, it will not be easy to develop greater willpower. Examining your concrete actions will help you start the transformation.
Make a list of the wrong habits you want to change. Start with small, gradual changes. Try to commit yourself to abandon an old behavior for a week, then continue making new changes slowly.

For example, you decide that after work, rather than watching a show, you will walk for 40 minutes. Commit to respecting your purpose for a week. In the following days, you can gradually increase the duration of the exercise, e.g. by walking for an hour.

On the occasions when the willpower is not yet sufficient, commit to bringing yourself back to the right path, even if it may mean having to be particularly hard on yourself. Doing so will help you understand that you are the only one who has the power to change your behavior.

Recognize and admit any failures. Register them on your food diary. Take responsibility for failure.

Describe the reasons that led to failure, highlighting your disappointment. For example, write something like, "At dinner, I ate dessert because I chose to, and I felt guilty after doing it." Although they may sound harsh words, many believe that saying them is useful to express clearly that they have failed. You will feel motivated to make greater efforts to be able to change.

For some, taking a weekly meal "out of the rules" can be a valid help to stay on track. A deprivation that has lasted too long may cause the whole project to go up in smoke. Sticking to a strict diet may seem more feasible when you know that at the end of the tunnel, you can give yourself the coveted food. If you think it might be useful to check you, consider scheduling a premium meal at the end of the week.

<u>Chapter Five</u>

Common Questions

Eating is a necessary activity—the body is like a car, and without fuel, it cannot work. Unfortunately, however, in our society, overloaded with food and obsessed with dieting, people build a relationship with extremely wrong foods, in which the act of eating becomes an automatic action and too often linked to negative emotions. In this chapter, I will try to explain to you what is the only thing you need to do to improve your relationship with food and make the act of eating an action that will not only bring nourishment but also pleasure.

Have you ever eaten food without even knowing what they are?

Do not worry; unfortunately, it happens to many people. Every day, people come to my studio to tell me how they respond unconsciously to their food stimuli, always repeating the same actions and, above all, feeling deprived of the strength to change.

They tell me how often they do not derive any joy from what they eat and, on the contrary, gain a lot of frustration or guilt from it, and they want to know what they can do to improve their relationship with food. They have often tried everything and feel tired and disappointed.

The solution is actually much simpler than what you may believe.

The only thing you need to do to improve your relationship

with food is not to do stressful diets (which only lower self-esteem) or spend whole days in the gym, but something much simpler: you have to become more aware of what you are doing.

Increasing awareness of your automated models can help you make more deliberate food choices and improve your relationship with food.

What you have to change is not so much the food you eat, but more on our relationship with it. Learning to eat with awareness will allow you to understand what your body really needs, and it will allow you to enjoy your meals.

In this way, in the end, you will reach your ideal weight without having to constantly resort to exasperating diets.

How do you do it?

Simple: you have to learn to be in contact with *you*! You have to ask yourself some good questions to help you become aware of the hundreds of food decisions you take every day without even realizing it.

Here are some good questions you must ask yourself to become more aware and improve your relationship with food.

1. Why do I eat?

This is the main question that will guide all your future decisions. And in the vast majority of cases, you do not know why you're eating! People hardly stop to wonder what drives them to go to the kitchen and open the pantry drawer. Many times, one believes that they are hungry, but in reality, they only feel like that in response to an emotional stimulus, such as boredom or stress. Learning to recognize this difference is the first step to effectively fight your urges and discover the real needs of your body. Take a break to ask yourself, "Am I really hungry?" Whenever you feel like you need to eat, it will help you differentiate your physical hunger from environmental and emotional stimuli.

2. When do I eat?

If you have ever followed a diet in your life, you will have realized that the traditional dietary approaches do nothing but provide you with a food plan where they tell you what you should eat, how much you have to eat, and what time you have to eat! This cannot be more wrong. These rules do nothing but disconnect you from your natural nourishment needs and only encourage you to ignore internal signals of hunger and satiety.

3. What do I eat?

Diets are definitely frustrating. They force you to eliminate a lot of things and often the best ones in terms of taste! To be able to do this, you are required a certain willpower that must be maintained for a very long time, which is very difficult even for the most persevering people. Learning to consume a little of everything in a moderate way, ranging from healthier foods to those that you eat for pleasure, will lead you to live your relationship with food in a much more balanced way. By freeing yourself from restrictions, you will develop the ability to respond to the wisdom of your body—that innate wisdom that is within each person.

4. How do I eat?

Quickly? Standing up? Watching TV? Many people eat this way and are so inclined to eat more—this feeling of satiety and satisfaction is, in fact, less when not paying attention to the food you introduce. Learn to avoid multitasking when you eat and dedicate quality time to the activity of eating. In this way, you will be able to feel what your body has to tell you, such as when it is time to stop, so as to avoid the binge you will later regret.

5. How much do you eat?

Normally, classic diets focus on how much you are allowed to eat using methods based on the control of calories or fat. This behavior, however, in the long run, leads you to spend an enormous amount of time, energy, and willpower. Turning the meal into a mechanical experience will make you disconnect from internal signals, and this will favor problematic behaviors rather than reducing them. Paying attention to the signs of satiety and determining small goals in the situation, such as feeling better after eating than before you start, will make you able to eat the "right" amount of food based on the real needs of your body. For example, young children eat when they are hungry and stop when they are full. They touch, smell, and explore food while eating it. Re-learning these innate behaviors in humans is essential for developing a healthy relationship with food.

<u>Chapter Six</u>

Three Meals a Day is a Social Construct.

Why do we eat what we eat? The answer suggested by common sense is that we choose to eat what we like. And it is a correct answer: satisfaction is the main factor influencing our food choices. But the question is more complex. Scientific literature has highlighted a link between food and the expression of both social and personal identity—we are what we eat, not only in biological terms but also in symbolic terms. In fact, food practices refer to the different collective belonging and manifest the individual adherence to a lifestyle. Moreover, social psychology, in explaining human behavior, takes into account the fact that we do not live in isolation but together with other people who inevitably influence us. Therefore, in addition to the tastes and information we possess (for example, on the presumed healthiness of certain foods), the influence of others also contributes to determining our eating habits, often through identification processes with different social groups. Without claiming to be exhaustive, let's look at some examples of social influence on eating behavior.

The first to influence us are certainly our parents, especially our mothers, who can condition us in different ways. First of all, through their example: our mothers are the first models we imitate, in general, and also with regard to the relationship with food. Secondly, our mothers even influence the development of our tastes because it circumscribes and delimits our experience with food: our mothers choose the one that enters the repertoire of the foods we come in contact with and selecting the foods to which we are exposed. When we were in their womb, we began to taste and learn about the flavors of our family and our culture. This selective exposure to food continues throughout the period of breastfeeding (even our mothers' milk takes the taste of what they eat) and continues for a long time. In fact, at least until the children reach 11-12 years old, our parents decide which foods come into the pantry and arrive at the table. This type of influence is fundamental because the selection of the food we are experiencing greatly influences our tastes, which are mainly formed through simple exposure and repeated experience. They are built on familiarity—we like what we are used to eating.

A second way by which tastes develop is through associations that are established between a certain food and a positive or negative situation. Parents can also influence these associations: if the family meal is a nice moment and an opportunity for sharing and living peacefully, our relationship with food will be connoted in a positive sense; if the meal is a battlefield, a place of conflict, in which they force us to eat something that does not go well, then our relationship with food will perhaps be compromised and will haunt us even into adulthood.

Growing up, our peers become increasingly important, both in general and as sources of influence, on our eating behaviour. Our peers influence us because we tend to imitate them. For example, at the end of a dinner with new friends, we often ask ourselves: "Should I get the dessert?" It may happen that we have a great desire for it, but if nobody takes it, we will probably give it up. Some research shows that people eat less if they are together with people who eat little and eat more if they are together with people who eat a lot. Why does this happen? In general, there are two fundamental reasons: on the one hand, if we do not know how to behave in a certain situation, which is perhaps new and unusual, we look at what others do to understand what is the appropriate behavior, and we repeat it; on the other hand, we imitate others because we identify with them because and we want to feel accepted or at least not seem strange or deviant. This is where the idea of having 3 meals a day came from. As we will see in the next chapter, however, it is *not* the best solution.

<u>Chapter Seven</u>

Established Intermittent Meal Plans

The recipe for living long and healthy would be to reduce protein intake: but what happens to our body with semi-fast regimes? According to Mark Mattson of the National Institute on Aging-Neuroscience, intermittent fasting generates a slight biological stress that pushes the body to reactivate its cellular defense against molecular damage. According to other experts, however, this would allow the body to detoxify, eliminating waste, toxins, and waste products.

Intermittent fasting is a flexible program and allows anyone with any kind of power to follow it. It is an effective way to lose body fat, to preserve lean mass, and to have energy throughout the fasting period.

Everyone knows what fasting is, but few people ever experience it.

Fasting is simply that time when you do not eat: usually, the longest time you do not eat is between dinner and breakfast, so that would be around 10 to 12 hours. It is no coincidence that the Anglo-Saxon countries use the word breakfast, which means "breaking a fast."

In detail, therefore, intermittent fasting (IF) is a diet that alternates phases of fasting (or underfeeding) long (from 16 to 36 hours) to feeding phases. It is simply adding a few hours to the night fast.

There are various methods: 16 hours of fasting and 8 of feeding at least 2 times a week, 16 hours of fasting and 8 of feeding every day, 24 hours of fasting 1 or 2 times a week (on the day of fasting, only one meal is eaten after 24 hours), 36 hours of fasting, and the Warrior diet (during the day, you can introduce very few calories from vegetables and/or dried fruit, and dinner only consists of just one meal).

When you follow this diet (if in good health and after consultation with your doctor), you may notice health benefits, including the decrease in body weight, decrease in blood glucose levels, increased lipolysis and fat oxidation, and decrease in stress related to food.

Is intermittent fasting good for everyone?

Intermittent fasting should not be followed by those who live the relationship with food in a nervous way, by those who cannot control the amount of food ingested, and by those who continually check the clock to know if they can start eating again.

Before making important choices from the point of view of food, you should always ask advice from an expert, primarily the family doctor—if you are in good health, and a specialist has given their consent, you can try the intermittent fasting road, perhaps starting a little at a time, grouping what you would eat during the whole day in an 8-hour band and fast the remaining 16. The goal must always be 16 hours, perhaps with the tolerance of one hour (15 to 17 hours). As always, before starting any diet or nutritional regiment, we advise you to see your doctor and discuss with him the new approach you want to take.

Why is fasting good?

As reported by Mark Mattson of the National Institute on Aging-Neuroscience, intermittent fasting provides a mild biological stress that drives the body to reactivate its cellular defense against molecular damage. Mice, for example, show higher levels of a protein that protects neurons from death. In this way, Mattson would argue that untimely fasting would remove the risk of stroke and cerebral decline, produce new neurons, and bring benefits to the whole body.

Fasting reduces inflammation, improves the immune system response, enhances the ability of cells to get rid of waste substances, slows the growth of tumors, and reduces the risk of heart disease. The thing that remains important, however, is to continue to drink lots of water. Fasting is not a low-calorie diet—a diet based on fruit or liquid. We do not consume fats, vitamins, or sugar; when you *really* fast, you do not eat anything at all.

In the body, autolysis is then started, which is essentially the process of destruction of worn out tissues. These tissues are replaced by new ones created by the same organism—in short, the body "eats itself" to regenerate itself. In addition to autolysis, fasting accelerates the cleansing of blood vessels, cells, and the environment in which they swim. So now that we have understood the basis of fasting, let's dive deeper into the topic and discover all the secrets of this modern way of eating.

Chapter Eight

Training and Fasting

For some time, there has been a total inversion with regard to the principles of weight loss and the basics of muscular anabolism.

Classic Approach

Food-induced Thermogenesis

The fundamentals of "traditional" dietetics suggest losing weight by exploiting also the specific dynamic action of food (ADS), or energy expenditure attributable to digestive, absorption, and metabolic processes.

In practice, with the same calories introduced, with increasing the division of meals, it is possible to burn more energy to process them. This allows you to reduce the amount of time "on an empty stomach" avoiding the "hunger" and keeping the metabolism speedy.

Cortisol and Thyroid Hormones

Some argue that this practice also favors the containment of an unwanted hormone, cortisol (also called "stress hormone") and maintenance of thyroid function (TSH and T3). Obviously, this system works as long as the caloric amount, the nutritional distribution, and the glycemic load-gauges of the meals are appropriate.

Preventing Catabolism

At the same time, in the context of muscle growth, it is (or was) a common opinion that to promote anabolism, it was necessary to "feed" continuously (and "as much as possible," avoiding the increase of fat) muscle fibrocells, in order to cancel any form of catabolism and promote proteosynthesis, *especially* thanks to the insulin stimulus.

What is Intermittent Fasting?

This principle is already heavily inflated and, to be sure, rather confused. It goes from the "caveman's diet," which involves a huge binge with one or two days of fasting, at the most reasoned "system 16/8" (where 16 is the hours of fasting and 8 is the hours in which 2 or 3 are consumed meals).

The cardinal principle of intermittent fasting is to create a fasting "window" (time lapse) with a duration that affects the overall caloric balance and hormone metabolism.

How Does It Work?

It seems that in conditions of food abstinence, in addition to a total insulin calm (remember that insulin is the parabolic hormone par excellence but also responsible for fat storage), there is a significant increase in another rather "interesting" hormone: l 'IGF-1 or somatomedin (some also mention an increase in testosterone).

The long deprivation of food is then responsible for the secretion of GH (somatotropin), also called "growth hormone" or, more sympathetically, "hormone of wellness." Unlike insulin, GH, while increasing hypertrophy, does not cause an adipose deposit, but the opposite! That is, it promotes the lipolysis necessary for weight loss. In practice, GH improves "all-around" body composition.

Always in bodybuilding, to increase muscle and decrease fat, it is essential to sequence the diet and training by pursuing distinctly first one and then the other goal. Today, since the intermittent fasting does result in an improvement of the body composition bilaterally (by increasing muscle mass and weight loss), it seems to be the only real solution to all problems.

Example:

Completely avoiding to cite bibliographic sources of dubious reliability (and seriousness), I will describe below the most interesting and undoubtedly best-suited variant that I could read.

First, I stress that despite using the fasting window, the remaining meals cannot be consumed freely. Moreover, to maximize the results of weight loss (and obviously those of increasing muscle mass), it is always necessary to perform the right physical activity.

The protocol differs in 3 daily meals and 1 training session with a fasting window equal to 16 hours.

- 1st meal to be eaten as soon as you rise up: a source of protein and carbohydrates with medium-low glycemic index; few fats
- 2nd meal – breakfast: complete
- Training (bodybuilding or high-intensity training)
- 3rd meal (to be done *immediately* after training) – lunch: complete

- Fasting window from 1:00 pm or 3:00 pm until the following morning.

Obviously, the system can be adapted to the lifestyle of the subject. I personally eat between 1pm and 6pm, using the mornings to do my workouts and cardio. I simply feel better not having any food in me while working, however; everyone is different though.

<u>Chapter Nine</u>

What Foods Can You Eat

Intermittent fasting is a diet based on the alternation of regular meals and fasting moments, with the aim of speeding up the metabolism and helping to lose weight faster. Here is an example of the benefits and the different patterns of the intermittent fasting diet.

Intermittent fasting is a diet based on the alternation of regular meals and moments of actual fasting. This type of on-off diet allows you to decide, according to different schemes, how to set the above alternation of normal meals and periods of pause from food, which would ensure a positive influence on the calorie balance and hormone metabolism, thus promoting fast weight loss and improving cardiovascular health and the immune system, in general. There are five main examples of intermittent fasting diet to choose from, in which time windows vary between fasting and normal meals, in essence.

Generally, in the examples of intermittent fasting diet, a split of the day is foreseen in two moments: a fasting phase called fast—which lasts several hours (from 12 to 19-20 hours), in which no food will be introduced with the exception of water, bitter coffee, tea and drinks without sugars—and another part called fed, in which you can eat regularly.

Intermittent Fasting: the 5 Examples of Fasting-based Diets

There are 5 main examples of a diet based on intermittent fasting. Here they are:

Intermittent Fasting or Intermittent Fasting Leangains

Devised by the athletic trainer Martin Berkhan, this method is based on scheme 16/8, i.e. the division of the day into two parts: 8 hours in which two or three meals can be consumed, and 16 hours of complete fasting.

Eat Stop Eat

This method was devised by the American nutritionist Brad Pilon, which consists of fasting for 24 hours for one or two days a week. In reality, however, in the off days, a normocaloric diet is allowed.

The Warrior Diet

This method, devised by Ori Hofmekler, provides a 4-hour fed phase—distributed between a dinner, where you can eat everything without any restriction of calories or macronutrient intake, and vegetable snacks rich in fiber and dried fruit.

The Fast Diet (or fasting every other day)

Based on the 5: 2 scheme, that is the possibility to eat regularly for 5 days a week and to make a strong calorie restriction in the other two days. In fact, in the off days, there is no actual fasting, but a maximum of 500 calories is allowed for women or 600 for men. The standard two-calorie menu should focus on a hearty breakfast—such as scrambled eggs, ham, and black tea— and a light dinner of fish or grilled chicken and vegetables. Lunch would be missed, while water and herbal teas are allowed throughout the day.

Whole Day Fasting

It is an Eat Stop Eat with one or two days of complete fasting, unlike the diet devised by Pilon. The good news is that in the other 5/6 days you can eat ad libitum (as you desire).

Intermittent fasting: What to Eat?

But what to eat in the fed phases of the various intermittent fasting diets?

Let us consider as the first example the most frequent type of intermittent fasting, which concentrates the fed phase in 8 hours, followed by a 16-hour fast. Here is a recommended-type menu:

Breakfast
Green tea, bitter coffee or herbal tea without sugar, water at will. (This phase is still fasting, considering that these drinks can be consumed safely even in the hours of fasting.)

Lunch (from 12 onwards)
Pasta with pesto, mixed vegetables with a spoon of oil, a fruit. (From here begins the fed phase, where you can have meals for the next 8 hours.)

Snack (from 16)
Dried fruit 15g, a fruit, 50g of rice or corn cakes

Dinner (at 19)
Baked cod, rye bread, mixed vegetables seasoned with a tablespoon of oil, a glass (125 mL) of wine. (Remember to stop the fed phase after 8 hours from the start of your first meal, breakfast excluded.)

This type of menu can also be followed for the 4 hours of fed Warrior Diet, to which is added the possibility of snacks based on vegetables rich in fiber and nuts—as well as for the two-day low-calorie diet Eat Stop Eat but trying to limit the doses, as they are days of reduction and semi-fasting to which they follow 5-6 wherein you can eat freely.

For the Whole Day Fasting Diet, there is no need for any indication, as unlike the previous ones where the fast is partial or relegated to some moments of the day, there are two days of absolute fasting per week, where you are only allowed to drink water, tea, and unsweetened drinks. For the others 5 days, there is no restriction.

Fast diet: what to eat in the 5:2 diet

Regarding the Fast diet, or diet every other day, based on the scheme 5:2, i.e. 5 days at full speed and 2 days at caloric restriction, the standard menu for the two days off provides a balance shared between an abundant breakfast and a light dinner that prefers protein foods.

Breakfast
Scrambled eggs, a thin slice of ham, and black tea

Dinner
Fish, chicken, and vegetables (all preferably grilled)
Water, herbal teas, or unsweetened green or black tea at will

Intermittent Fasting: When to Avoid It?

Although it is not such a drastic diet, intermittent fasting is not suitable for everyone. It is, in fact, not recommended for people suffering from diabetes, hypoglycemia, and cortisol imbalance.

It is also best to avoid it if you are subject to chronic fatigue or being pregnant or breastfeeding.

What to Eat in Intermittent Fasting: Guidelines

To make the most of your calorie intake on a day of fasting:

1) Choose more protein meals that help you feel full longer. Because proteins have enough calories, you cannot take unlimited amounts to reach the maximum limit set by your fasting day, which is 500 calories. However, you can still make proteins the main source of calories.

2) Fill the dish with low-calorie vegetables. They give a sense of satiety, are tasty, and are good for the health. Cook with steam, bake with a teaspoon of oil, or sauté in the pan. Then, add some spices or flavorings to prepare a tasty meal. You can also choose to eat raw salad.

3) Keep the carbohydrates to a minimum: they are rich in calories and make you feel hungry quickly. Among the high-carbohydrate foods, you should avoid potatoes, sweet potatoes, pasta, rice, bread, some fruits (bananas, grapes, melons, prunes, raisins, dates, and other nuts), breakfast cereals, fruit juices, corn-sole-panicle/sweet corn, and anything containing sugar or other syrups.

4) Do not be afraid of fat: although fat is rich in calories, it helps you feel full. Include small amounts of fat in the fasting meal.

Although the recommended caloric intake is 500 calories for women and 600 calories for men, it is not necessary to be really so stiff—but it will be necessary to weigh or measure at least the high-calorie ingredients in your recipes and calculate the calories to avoid overeating the allowed threshold.

A prepared meal can be a solution without too many problems. As with home-cooked meals, look for options that are low in carbohydrates and sugars and rich in protein and vegetables.

What to eat after fasting?

Intermittent fasting is the best way to eat for food lovers! In the days of not fasting, you are free to eat whatever you want, generally speaking.

Although, of course, if you want to lose weight, maybe you'll have to limit yourself to eating whatever you want. **Additionally, as strange as it may seem, the days where you do not fast probably will help you reduce your appetite instead of increasing it.**

You may find that you are not very hungry the day after fasting. You do not need to eat much if you do not want to. It is advisable, instead, to wait to feel the stimulus of hunger before eating on a day when you are not fasting.

Your tastes can change so as to no longer feel the desire for sweet and sugary foods.

You will understand hunger better, and you will feel less the desire to eat snacks. Then, you can develop the ability to wait for meals without worrying about when it will be time to eat.

This kind of changes will not happen immediately: your hunger on non-fasting days can vary greatly. You may find that you are really hungry and eat a lot on the days when you do not fast.

Many people experience this in the early days.

Do not worry if this happens; focus only on following your scheduled fasts.

After 6 weeks of fasting, if you still have hunger problems and cannot limit yourself to food and therefore are not losing weight, you may decide to change the method of fasting or make other changes. You should aim to eat normally on days when you are not fasting.

The joy of intermittent fasting is that you can spend most of your free time on food anxiety while controlling your weight and living healthily.

Some people limit their calories on days when they do not fast in an attempt to accelerate weight loss. Although this may work in the short term, it's probably not a good idea in the long run.

If you do not have your normal feeding days, you will probably feel deprived of your favorite foods and develop "diet fatigue."

If intermittent fasting has to become your way of life, it is important that you do it sustainably for a long time.

Chapter Ten

Sample Meal Ideas

Intermittent Fasting Food Plan

The intermittent fasting food plan by Ori Hofmekler is based on a very simple and intuitive structure:

Phase 1 - Under Power (for about 20 hours)

During the first part of the day, few foods are allowed—mostly of plant origin, such as seeds and simple proteins, i.e. all foods that are not very demanding for our digestive system. This is intended to facilitate detoxification of the body.

The prolonged (but controlled) state of under-feeding triggers physiological processes such as increased insulin sensitivity and increased production of anabolic hormones to counteract the state of "resource shortage" and to make the most of the few present.

Phase 2 – Supercharging (for the remaining 4 hours)

After Phase 1, the body finds itself *emptied* of resources and in a condition of maximum sensitivity to nourishment.

This particular condition makes sure that a large amount of nutrients introduced during supercharging is not lost or "stored" as fat (also due to the low level of insulin).

During this phase, there is no particular constraint on the type of food to be taken or its quantity.

Of course, taking on a diet like this also requires a team of specialists to follow you on the way, since you must not forget that you are a unique biological entity, and as such you will have individual responses that will need specific adjustments to allow optimization of the diet without incurring problems of any kind.

If some types of food programs are intuitive because they involve phases of total fasting in phases in which you can eat anything, in other cases indications are needed.

Take for example the leangains diet which, as mentioned, provides a fed phase of 8 hours, and a fast phase of 16 hours.

At breakfast and throughout the day you can give yourself green tea, bitter coffee, unsweetened teas, water.

At lunch, instead, after 12, you can eat pasta with pesto, mixed vegetables with a tablespoon of oil, fruit. (From here begins the fed phase, where you can have meals for the next 8 hours)

From 4 pm, you can have a snack with 15 g of dried fruit, a fruit and 50 g of rice or corn cakes.

At dinner, after 7 pm, the program includes baked cod, rye or wholemeal bread, mixed vegetables seasoned with a tablespoon of oil, a glass of wine. It is important to stop the fed phase, after 8 hours from the start of the first meal, excluding breakfast.

The fast diet consists of 5 days in which you eat regularly and 2 days of caloric restriction. In these 2 days the consumption of protein foods is recommended. At breakfast, you can eat for example, scrambled eggs, ham and tea; for dinner, instead, chicken, fish and grilled vegetables.

The most frequent type of intermittent fasting is leangains, which concentrates the fed phase in 8 hours, followed by a 16-hour fast. Below we propose an example of a menu, which must however be modified according to the different needs:

Breakfast: green tea, bitter coffee or herbal tea without sugar, water at will. This phase is still fasting;

Lunch: wholemeal pasta, mixed vegetables with a tablespoon of oil, a fruit. From here begins the fed phase;

Snack: dried fruit, a fruit, rice cakes or corn or a low-fat yogurt; **Dinner**: meat and lean fish baked or grilled, tofu or seitan, rye or wholemeal bread, mixed vegetables seasoned with a tablespoon of oil. This is the last phase of fed.

It is important to stop the fed phase after 8 hours from the start of your first meal (breakfast excluded since you consume only liquids). So, for example, if you eat lunch at 12 you can eat until 8pm.

Additional Resources

Here is a collection of studies that can help you better understand the concepts discussed in the book:

https://www.ncbi.nlm.nih.gov/pmc/articles/PMC3680567/

https://www.ncbi.nlm.nih.gov/pmc/articles/PMC4403246/

https://www.health.harvard.edu/blog/intermittent-fasting-surprising-update-2018062914156

https://newatlas.com/intermittent-fasting-16-8-diet-study-science/55105/

https://newatlas.com/intermittent-fasting-causes-diabetes-debate/54685/

https://www.healthline.com/nutrition/intermittent-fasting-guide

https://www.businessinsider.com/intermittent-fasting-diet-health-benefits-weight-loss-2018-6

https://www.johnshopkinshealthreview.com/issues/spring-summer-2016/articles/are-there-any-proven-benefits-to-fasting

https://sciencebasedmedicine.org/intermittent-fasting/

https://thedoctorweighsin.com/what-science-has-to-say-about-intermittent-fasting/

https://www.popsci.com/intermittent-fasting-science

<u>Conclusion</u>

The next step is to stop reading and to start doing whatever it is that you need to do in order to ensure that you are able to create amazing intermittent fasting recipes and dishes. If you find that you still need help getting started, you will likely have better results by creating a schedule that you hope to follow—including strict deadlines for various parts of the tasks as well as the overall completion of your preparations.

Studies show that complex tasks that are broken down into individual pieces, including individual deadlines, have a much greater chance of being completed when compared to something that has a general need of being completed but no real timetable for doing so. Even if it seems silly, go ahead and set your own deadlines for completion—complete with indicators of success and failure. After you have successfully completed all your required preparations, you will be glad you did. For example, you can think about practicing one new intermittent fasting food habit every day, before becoming a general master of the diet. It is your choice, and it is the beauty of dieting and cooking.

Once you have tried the same recipe many times, it is the right moment to invite your friends and ask them to try the intermittent fasting diet—they are going to love it and, best of all, see incredible results with it.

<u>Book Two</u>

The Carnivore Diet

Eat Meat to Quickly Lose Fat,
Lean Out and Cleanse Your Body.

*Includes Meal Plans to Get You Started
Today*

Michael D Kaiser

Receive free alerts for Carnivore Diet meal plans and testimonials

www.CarnivoreCleanse.com

Table of Contents

Introduction

This book is based on someone that decided to try the Carnivore Diet plan after not being able to burn off the remaining sub-cutaneous layer of fat, even though he was exercising intensely, lifting weights, doing fasting and high intensity training, eating clean and healthy, etc.

When the author tried the meat only diet for 7 days, he was very afraid of health repercussions or developing high cholesterol. But NONE of that happened, in fact his cholesterol went down 7 points and his energy ZOOMED, and his abs finally showed after only 7 days, plus working out routinely as well. Previously he was on a mostly vegan diet. The author decided that the carnivore diet is really great for resetting the body metabolism and health, almost like a cleanse if you want to use that term.

There are great benefits to eating whole plant-based foods, but for some people it is not enough; if you are one of these people, the Carnivore Diet may be great for you to reset or even switch over to long term. The key is to eat only WHOLE meats, not processed meats.

The following chapters will discuss the carnivore diet and everything that it entails. Like most people, you probably do not think it is possible to survive, thrive and receive health benefits on a meat-only diet. Yet there are numerous people doing exactly that.

There are numerous instances in history when civilizations survived on nothing else but meat diets only. There are numerous studies from around the world that showcase how communities live and thrive on the carnivore diet.

This book will teach all you need to know about the carnivore diet, what it entails and why you may want to follow this diet. You will also learn how to begin this diet, why it is a stress-free diet and what benefits you will gain.

Some of the biggest health benefits that seem to come from eating meat only are fat loss, increased metabolism, significantly increased feelings of wellness and energy. Why this occurs has a lot to do with how the body processes WHOLE meat (not processed meat or junk chemically altered meat). We are going to explore how you can start experimenting with this "diet' if you are at an end-roads with your current plan that is not working for you (Fat loss, low energy, losing sub-cutaneous fat, etc..)

<u>Chapter One</u>

What is the Carnivore Diet?

There are plenty of diets and nutrition trends instructing us on the best way to eat. One of the latest is the carnivore diet. This is a pretty simple diet with a simple equation. The equation largely summarizes the diet.

Meat + Water = Carnivore Diet

Introduction to the Carnivore Diet

The carnivore diet is a diet that requires the consumption of only animal food and avoiding everything else.

This diet protocol calls for restricting your carbohydrate intake and eliminate plat food intake completely. It is the direct opposite of a vegan diet but closely resembles the keto diet. Both the carnivore and keto diets rely heavily on proteins and fats as the main source of energy.

The carnivore diet allows you to eat meat and products derived from animals. For instance, you can have fish, beef, meats, eggs, and products such as cream and butter and al other dairy products. However, the diet protocol requires you to avoid other food types like grains, vegetables, nuts, fruits, and seeds.

Complete opposite of a vegan diet

The carnivore diet is a complete opposite of the vegan diet. Science has, for decades, steered us towards pursuit of plant based diets for optimum health and well being while discouraging us from heavy consumption of meats. However, there have been plenty of positive attributes from people following this diet. There are reports from numerous individuals about the health benefits of eating as required by this protocol.

The positive feedback from numerous reports of individuals who've tried this diet has prompted even more people to try it out. The results have been impressive so fat. Some of the positive attributes from people who've tried this diet include faster weight loss, mental clarity, healthier digestive system and improved athletic performance.

The carnivore diet has a simple approach that makes it attractive to anyone searching for a diet that does not come with any complicated nutrition tactics like calculating calories and macros, timing your meals, and so on. The simplicity of this diet and the good reports coming in have made this diet attractive thus far. All that you need to do is to as per this diet is to eat animal foods including beef, fish, eggs, and dairy. You should also stay away from all other foods.

Foods you Should Avoid

Carbohydrates: You need to ensure that you do not take any carbohydrates. These are apparently restricted from the carnivore diet.

Vegetables: You are not supposed to take have vegetables with your diet.

Supplements: you should not take any dietary supplements. The reason for this is that the carnivore diet contains all the minerals and nutrients that the body requires in order to thrive.

Foods you should Eat

Dairy: Dairy is a product derived from animals. It includes diet items like cheese, butter, and milk. You will find, however, that most carnivore dieters prefer to skip dairy or limit its intake due to lactose intolerance that develops in the course of the diet.

Fish: All types of fish are allowed but especially those with lots of fat content. These include fish species like salmon, haddock, and halibut. Seafood is also generally acceptable.

Animal fat products: You can include animal fat products with your diet. These products include tallow, lard, and others so as to enhance your calorie intake.

Meat: You are generally allowed to consume all types of meats. These include red meat, fatty cuts, beef, steak, and all others. These are basically the staples of the carnivore diet.

Since carbohydrates are not part of your diet, then you should ensure that you receive the bulk of your nutrition intake from meats.

Meat products

- o Steaks – sirloin, chuck eye, ribeye, strip
- o Ground beef
- o Animal internal organs (optional)
- o Roast – chick, prime rib, brisket

Organ meats: There are some carnivore dieters who are of the opinion that organ meats are essential. The reasoning here is that evidence exists that shows organs aid in the development of human brain. However, not every carnivore dieter is of this opinion. Many prefer taking fish oils, especially oils from cold water fishes like cod. Ideally, you should consider adding cold water fish, liver, and brains to your diet. All these are rich in DHA which is an essential fatty acid. DHA has a vital role in proper functioning of the brain.

Additional Meats

- o Lamb – lamb chops, shank, ribs
- o Pork – shoulder, pork belly, butt roasts, ribs
- o Poultry – wings, drumsticks, thighs, chicken breasts
- o Fish – trout, crab, sardines, mackerel, scallops, shrimp, lobster

Beverages

- o Bone broth
- o Water – with minerals and carbonation or without
- o Tea

o   Coffee

Coffee is generally regarded as a plant extract. Some carnivore dieters opt to do without it while others freely have it. If you are generally a coffee drinker, then you are free to keep on taking it. Some strict adherents of this diet urge gradual withdrawal. When it comes to meats, you should focus more on grass feed meat and avoid the processed kind. The latter contains additives and preservatives that you do not want in your diet.

How much should you eat?

Basically, you are required to eat as much food as you can. You should eat until you are completely full and whenever you feel hungry. The mantra is to listen to your body and follow what it says.

o   Listen to your body
o   Eat at least two meals per day, more if possible
o   Let your appetite guide you

Even as your body heals and adapts, after years, possibly decades, of malnutrition, you can expect to start eating twice as much as before once your body heals completely. The general guide is to have between two and four ounces of fatty meat each day. Try not to restrict your calorie or food intake and force fasting. This is not part of the carnivore diet and is discouraged.

How do carnivore dieters eat?

A majority of dieters, up to 70%, eat two meals per day. About 10% eat three meals each day while only 20% have 1 meal per day. Ideally, though, you should not count the number of meals that you have in a day. Instead, you should focus on eating whenever you feel hungry and eat until you are full.

Snacks: If you eat sufficient meats throughout the day, then you will probably not see the need to snack during the day. Should you feel hungry then you should increase your meals and eat more during each meal.

Some people tend to snack and do so even when they do not feel hungry. If you really have to snack, then think about pork rinds. Make sure that any meats you eat are not cooked in vegetable fat. In due course, you will realize that most snacking will go away.

A Very Simple Diet

The carnivore diet is one of the simplest diets out there. It encourages you to consume meat only. You do not need to count calories or time your meals. All you need to focus on is eating whenever you feel hungry and eat as much meat as you want. Here is a look at a simple carnivore meal plan.

Breakfast: Bacon with scrambled eggs and tea or black coffee

Lunch: Lamb chops or a t-bone steak

Supper: Porterhouse or 80/20 grass-fed beef

Carnivore Basic Food List

- o Unprocessed meat: steak, red meat, fatty meat products
- o Fish: especially the oily and fatty kinds like sardines and salmon

- o Whole eggs
- o Bone marrow
- o Bone broth
- o Fatty meat products
- o Dairy
- o condiments

The ideologies of the carnivore diet are based largely on those of the ketogenic diet. There are studies showing that people who eat carbs daily are 30% likely too die compared to those who do not. The same studies showed that those who consume a high fat diet have a 23% less chance of dying compared to those who consume less fat. The study was conducted by researchers at McMaster University.

It is credible studies like these coupled with positive outcomes from dieters that are convincing more and more people to take up the carnivore dieting lifestyle. Take Dr, Anthony Gustin, for instance who is the Perfect Keto Diet founder. Dr.

Gustin's current diet consists of 90% carnivore. He carried out a 30-day experiment and realized his body could stay in ketosis even as he ate meats only.

Chapter Two

The History of the Carnivore Diet

We have been taught ever since we were young that regular meat consumption is fattening, unhealthy, heart-attack inducing, artery clogging, tumor producing, and cholesterol raising and constipating food that should be avoided as much as possible. We were made to believe that a diet full of vegetables and generally plant-based is the most ideal diet on the planet for optimum health.

There is no time in history where human population was confined to a plant-based diet. Neither is there a civilization that depended entirely on a vegan diet. However, there are numerous examples in history of communities that have existed largely on meat-based diets for generations and generations. These families that largely ate meat were never sickly or unhealthy compared to the general populations.

The communities of real people having mostly meat diet for extended periods of time provide us with a lot of insights and powerful information into this diet. We get to learn more about meats and their implications on our bodies and health compared to traditional scientific studies. Conventional scientific studies focus on a small group of individuals for a limited period of time.

Carnivorous Ancestors

If we take a closer look at the diets of our ancestors, we find that there are numerous examples of communities and populations across varied geographical regions and ethnic backgrounds that have opted for a carnivore diet across multiple generations. Here is a look at some examples of communities that practiced a largely carnivorous diet throughout history.

- Maasai from East Africa who consume mainly milk and meat
- Nomads living in Mongolia who lived largely on dairy and meat
- The Sioux of South Dakota ate mostly buffalo meat
- Canadian Inuits whose diet consists largely of fish, whale, seal and walrus
- Gaucho Brazilians who eat mostly meat and beef products
- Russian arctic Chukotka who existed on caribou, fish, and marine animals

Not only did these communities survive on largely meat diets, they thrived. Most of them displayed exceptional strength and health. For instance, the Eskimos from Point Hope ate mostly meat diet consisting of sea cultures, whale, and walrus. According to research, their diet consisted of 35% protein and 50% animal fat.

The researchers discovered that the Point Hope Eskimos had ten times less incidences of heart disease compared to the general population across America. Also, their levels of bad cholesterol were much lower compared to their Caucasian counterparts across continental America.

The Eskimos

Think about the Eskimos, for instance. They had no chance of eating fruit or vegetable any time of the year. Animals such as seals contain zero fiber. By all means, these Eskimo communities ate virtually no vegetables nor fruits. They never tilled the land not harvested crops. Yet they are much healthier than your average person.

While their diets are low in fiber, they are high in animal fat and protein. Such diets generally scare the average American and even institutions like the American Cancer Society, Harvard School of Public Health, and the USDA. Most of these institutions oppose carnivore diets and the consumption of high fat and high protein diets.

A lot of people are puzzled as to how these carnivorous populations obtained their minerals and vitamins without eating any fruits or colorful vegetables. Many wonder how come these communities do not suffer from heart conditions, diabetes, gout, cancers, and other chronic conditions.

To be able to understand how the carnivore diet works, it is advisable to examine closely two different groups of people whose information is readily available. By studying these two groups, it is possible to make some crucial yet fascinating findings relating to the carnivore versus regular diets.

Arctic Communities vs. East African Herdsmen

The Arctic communities live mostly in Alaska, Greenland, Russia, and Canada. The diets of these communities started to change some time in the early 1900s when trade routes and travelers begun introducing foods such as flour, dairy products and flour. These foods did not exist prior to these new trade routes.

In East Africa, we have herdsmen like the Maasai, Samburu, and Pokot. They live around the equator where the temperatures are quite high. According to traditions, the males in these communities lived on only animal products, mostly dairy products and meat. This they do for a period of at least 14 years when the boys turn 28 and become warriors. Teams of American researchers descended into these communities to try and figure out why they were in such exceptional health despite their "unhealthy" diets.

Point Hope in Alaska is a pretty remote location where residents consume a mostly carnivorous diet due to its isolated status. This region was also the subject of a close study by scientists from America. According to the research findings, communities living at this remote location, their diet consisted mostly of walrus and whale meat. An average adult consumed about 3,000 calories per day. Of these 3,000 calories, about 35% was obtained from protein sources while at least 50% was from fat. Carbohydrate intake was limited to about 15 – 20%. This was largely in the form of animal starch or glycogen. The only sugar they had was a type of sucrose sugar that was primarily used to sweeten coffee or tea.

Arctic Findings

Studies were conducted more recently on southwestern Alaskan natives who consumed less traditional foods and more vegetables than their remote counterparts. However, according to the findings of the study, the Alaskans pursuing a traditional diet with more fat and proteins had lower triglyceride levels compared to their southwestern counterparts whose diet consists largely of vegetables and grains with less meat and fat.

Even as recently as the 1980s, very few deaths among the Greenland Eskimos is attributed to heart conditions yet the majority of residents live beyond 60 years of age. There are reports of arctic residents with artery-cholesterol buildup. However, these residents are identified as those who consume a combination of both traditional and modern diets. The high life expectancy of the Eskimos and residents of the arctic is attributed largely to the absence of heart conditions and low cholesterol levels.

Africa Findings

Findings among the African tribes existing largely on a carnivore diet indicate that heart diseases are completely unheard of. Research scientists examined over 600 subjects who were Maasai males. Most of them were 40 years and above. According to this study, only one participant had ever experienced a heart attack. The researchers then examined the hearts of 50 dead Maasai men and found that none of them had passed away due to coronary diseases. Just as with the Eskimos, there was the presence of some cholesterol and fat deposits in some blood vessels but none were serious enough to raise the alarm or cause a blockage.

Among the African communities existing on a carnivore diet, most of the men acquired over 66% of their daily calorie intake from eating animal fat. They consumed about 600 mg of cholesterol and 300 grams of fat each day. Nutritionists and dieticians advise us today to keep our fat intake to between 25 – 35% of our calorie intake and keep out cholesterol amounts to 300 mg per day or less. This means that the African communities were consuming more than twice the recommended amounts without suffering any health consequences.

Effect of Meat on Blood Pressure

Residents of Greenland often consumed a diet rich in animal fat, fish, and meats with very few fruits, dairy products, or vegetables. Sometime in the 1980s and 1990s, some of these people migrated to Denmark and consumed diets high in grains, vegetables, fruits, and other plant products. After a while, researchers discovered that the migrants, now consuming a normal diet, had blood pressure that was 10 points higher than their counterparts back in Greenland.

This was puzzling because they drank less, smoked less, and even weighed a lot less compared to their Greenland counterparts. The crucial point that you need to note here is that consuming less meat while eating more vegetables and fruits, as we are always advised to do, does not necessarily protect or improve health, especially when it comes to blood pressure.

Blood pressure among the East African Maasai

Among the east African nomadic tribes of the Maasai and others, it was discovered by researchers that males aged 15 to 55 averaged a blood pressure of 120/80. It is only about 1% of males who had any significant blood pressure levels that would be of concern. The average weight of the nomadic males was 134 while the average height was 5 foot 7 inches.

The Great Puzzle

It is worth noting then, that communities living off eating meat with plenty of cholesterol and saturated fats are healthy with no weight, blood pressure, or heart problems. Apparently, saturated fats, meats, and cholesterol should be major causes of numerous chronic conditions. On the other hand, vegetables, fruits, and grains protect us from heart conditions and high blood pressure.

So the question is why do communities consuming so much meat, saturated fats and oils fair much better than those consuming supposedly healthier diets consisting of vegetables, fruits, grains, and nuts? While there are no concrete or scientific answers to this and other pertinent questions, it is crucial to note the discrepancy and think about it.

How the Carnivore Diet Works

Animal products like meats are naturally zero carb. This means they do not contain any carbohydrates. When carbohydrate is restricted in our diets, then we lose the need for some nutrients. Also, the vitamins necessary for carbohydrate metabolism become redundant.

A good example is vitamin A. according to a study that focused on this vitamin, it was discovered that in the absence of carbohydrates in the diet, this vitamin was no longer necessary for metabolism regulation. Basically, when we eliminate carbs from the diet, the body will find an alternative source of energy. When this happens, it will enter a phase known as ketosis. In this instance, fat within the body will be converted for energy use. It is thought the body would much rather source its energy from fats via ketosis than any other source. In fact, there are several benefits to the body when ketosis becomes the main source of energy. The carnivore diet operates in an almost similar manner to the keto diet. However, there are some notable differences. Let us examine some of these differences closely.

Difference between Carnivore Diet and Keto Diet

There are some stark similarities between the keto and carnivore diets. For instance, they both allow regular consumption of proteins and fats while eliminating carbohydrates.

However, the carnivore diet is considered to be a lot more restrictive and takes matters a step further compared to the ketogenic diet. For instance, the keto diet allows you to consume a fair amount of non-animal fatty foods like avocados, coconut oil, and nuts as well as large quantities of plant foods like vegetables.

The ketogenic diet focuses more on high fat and moderate protein intake in order to enable the body enter the ketosis state and start using ketones as the main source of energy for the body. However, the carnivore diet prohibits the intake of other types of fats except animal fat.

Also, the carnivore diet has no macronutrient requirements compared to diets such as keto. However, through this diet, you will still be able to reach ketosis which will be the body's main source of energy.

The keto diet requires you to take 5 – 10% carbohydrates, 20 – 30% proteins, and 60 – 70% fat. In comparison, the carnivore diet has got no such requirements. You do not need to measure or count calories. All you are required to do is eat as much meat as you can until you are full. You are also required to eat whenever you feel hungry but are not restricted to eating only during specified meal times.

There are some dairy foods that are not allowed as part of the ketogenic diet mainly due to higher carbs content. However, in the carnivore diet, all dairy products are permitted because they are derived from animals. The carnivore diet allows all dairy and meat products from animals. These are the main differences between the keto diet and the carnivore diet. However, there are also plenty of similarities.

Adapting to the carnivore diet

The body requires some time before it can adapt to the carnivore diet. Keep in mind that different people have different metabolic rates. Our bodies need to adjust from getting their energy from one source to another. With most people, it takes between two and three weeks for the change to be effective. This is also the same time it takes the average person to start enjoying the benefits of this eating pattern. Those, such as athletes, who have primarily been used to carbs as the main source of energy end up taking much longer to adjust, like three weeks.

Reasons Why Vegetables, Grains, and Fruits are not Allowed

Meat is not necessarily easier to digest but is more nutrient-dense and compact compared to plant matter. Herbivore diet is much more efficient at extracting nutrients. However, such a diet requires that you eat and keep on eating a lot of the time. This is seen in a lot of herbivores. Herbivores have very long digestive systems. A meat only diet does not require you to eat so much throughout the day.

Most vegetables contain toxic enzymes that kill most of the nutrients. This is a self-defense mechanism that most vegetables possess. As a result, you will not get as much nutrients from vegetables because of this. On the other hand, nutrition from meat sources is readily available. You will therefore receive more nutrition from a carnivore diet compared to a herbivore diet consisting of vegetables, grains, and fruits.

<u>Chapter Three</u>

Getting Started with the Carnivore Diet

According to research findings, the carnivore diet is really worth your while. It may sound a little different from what you are used but it actually works. There is plenty of anecdotal testimony out there that supports this way of eating. This is probably why there is a growing shift by conscious individuals including health dieters, athletes, and numerous others towards this way of life.

The main reason why people make the shift to the carnivore diet is because of its numerous benefits. Among these benefits, significant weight loss, an increase in focus and improved moods rank very high with dieters. These are the reasons why this diet is very popular across America and beyond. The carnivore diet also has numerous principles that are very similar to those of a high fat, low carb keto diet. This is also another reason why it is compelling to others. Basically, a diet that restricts your carbohydrate intake is one that is great for you.

Essential Preparation

Before you get started with the carnivore diet, you need to prepare yourself psychologically and physically. A lot of people experiment with this diet for various reasons so it is crucial that you determine why you wish to pursue this eating lifestyle. Let us examine some of the reasons why people choose this diet over all others.

1. Mood: conditions such as depression, focus, bipolar, brain fog and so on

2. Gastro-Intestinal: digestive conditions such as gas, bloating, colitis, heartburn, and gastric reflux

3. Autoimmune disease: conditions like migraines, arthritis, asthma, Lyme's disease, multiple sclerosis and numerous others

4. Keto benefits: benefits like muscle gain, weight loss, and many more

5. Skin conditions: helps with conditions such as acne, rosacea, eczema, psoriasis

Questions

Most people often have questions and doubts about this diet. This is normal and is to be expected. Some of the questions people ask are indicated below.

- o How come people on the carnivore diet do not suffer scurvy?
- o Can you have proper bowel movements with no fiber?
- o What about all the cholesterol?
- o Won't this diet surely lead to chronic coronary conditions?
- o I will probably end up with cancer, right?

The Adaptation Period

Different people transition differently into the carnivore or all-meat diet. If you were on a keto diet or the HFLC (high fat low carb) diet, then you transition will be easy because your body is probably in keto.

However, if you are transitioning from the standard American diet or SAD which is high in carbohydrates, then it becomes quite difficult to adapt. You should expect some mild challenges during this transition period.

The discomfort that you will experience during the transition period is simply your body's reaction to carbohydrate withdrawal as well as elimination of certain additives, coloring, and chemicals found in processed foods.

Symptoms during Transition

- o Metallic or bad taste in mouth
- o Headaches, brain fog, dizziness
- o Bad breath, bad smells, irritability
- o Digestive issues, sore throat, chills
- o Diarrhea, nausea, soreness, sugar cravings
- o Muscle aches, poor performance, low energy
- o Night sweats, insomnia, rapid heart rate
- o Nocturia or frequent urination at night

What causes all these symptoms?

You may wonder what is going on with your body during the transition period. One of these is something known as fluid rebalancing. The first thing that happens when you cut out carbs is that your insulin levels fall drastically. Once these levels are significantly low, a signal is sent to the kidneys requesting the release of sodium from the body.

You will probably lose about 10 pounds of water in just a couple of days because the water will follow the sodium. The remaining glycogen in your body will eventually be converted into glucose before the body eventually switches to using fatty acids.

From sugar to fat for energy

The body will then begin the transition process from burning mostly glucose for energy to fat. This process needs the body to make a lot of adjustments. Most of these will rely on your metabolic flexibility. This term refers to your body's ability to handle varied sources of energy. People who are accustomed to consuming most carbohydrates will experience feelings similar to withdrawal symptoms like drug addicts do, for instance.

Hormone rebalancing

You are also likely to experience hormonal rebalance and response to the changes take place especially with your metabolism. One of the most significant hormones affected is the T3 thyroid hormone. This hormone is responsible for metabolism, regulation of body temperature, and heart rate. It is also very closely aligned to carbohydrates.

Cortisol plays an important role in the body. For instance, it helps in managing inflammation and is involved in regulating blood sugar levels. Cortisol will be released into the bloodstream as you begin the transition process especially when you start craving sugars and carbs.

During this entire process, the body is actually getting rid of addictions to all the unhealthy carbs and sugars. As the addictions disappear, there will be other changes in your body as well. For instance, you are likely to experience changes in the way the brain transmits signals to your stomach.

This communication channel between your gut and the brain greatly influences a lot of other aspects including neurotransmitters like serotonin and dopamine as well as hormones. These tend to have a huge impact on matters like addictions, cravings, and moods. Going through symptoms akin to withdrawal is not uncommon so you can expect this to happen to you.

Commitment

When you decide you are going to follow this lifestyle, then you should be prepared to make a commitment otherwise it will not work out. Basically, if you are unable to fully commit yourself, then you should wait until such a time as when you will eventually be ready. This may probably be in the form of a condition or possibly a burning desire. Some people on the other hand tend to give up at the slightest sign of discomfort. You should expect a transition period of two weeks or less when your body makes the necessary adjustment.

Prepare for the Transition Period

If you get organized, then you will be able to minimize and even eliminate this transition stage and its numerous symptoms.

You should be prepared

It is crucial that you prepare yourself for this process. Being mentally prepared is definitely advisable so accept and understand the symptoms that you expect to encounter. Once you are mentally prepared, you can also then get physically prepared.

Start eating lots of meat

One of the reasons why you may suffer the symptoms mentioned above is under-eating. Plenty of people do not eat enough because they related this eating lifestyle to other dietary lifestyles that limit food intake. Remember to eat as much meat as you feel like, or to satisfaction, without restricting intake or tracking macronutrients.

Hydrate throughout the day

The carnivore diet needs you to drink plenty of water throughout the day. As a rule, you need to drink water equivalent to half your bodyweight in ounces. For instance, if you weight 120 pounds, then you need to drink 60 ounces of water each day. Do this especially during the adaption stage. Once the adaption stage is over and you have settled down into this eating style, you should only drink whenever you feel thirsty. Basically you will only drink water when you want to.

Supplement your electrolytes

Another step that you need to follow is to supplement your electrolytes. As your body loses water, you also lose plenty of electrolytes. These include chloride, magnesium, potassium, and sodium. Supplementing is therefore a step that you should take. If you need to supplement, then think about the Pink Himalayan rock salt. It is an excellent source of chloride and sodium. In most cases this should be enough. However, you can also supplement with magnesium and potassium.

You can take supplements that are popular with meat-only dieters. One of these is Ionic Potassium. Alternatively, you can drink meaty bone broth on a regular basis. Bone broth will provide you with lots of the minerals you need including sodium and potassium.

Expect some problem bowel movement

You can expect to encounter gastro-intestinal problems. Apparently these are quite common and mostly for those originally on a low fat diet. Your gall bladder might experience some challenges making the transition. One solution to this problem is choosing lean cuts of meat with very little fat. This is however not a really great idea for a carnivore dieter so follow the solution only for the short term.

Since you are likely to experience bowel movement challenges, you should supplement your diet in this regard. Take a lipase supplement a couple of minutes before your meals. It will help ease your bowel movement challenges and improve your bathroom experience.

If you are coming from a low fat diet, then you might need to take ox bile with your meals in order to ease bowel movement. Sometimes low stomach acid levels can cause problems and you could suffer GERD. Find a supplement to help ease the gastric reflux such as Betaine HCL. This one works really great where others may not be so effective.

Alternatively, you may also consider removing rendered fat from your meats once cooked. Rendered fat is the liquid fat that is produced during cooking. If you notice, in due course of time, that your bowel movements are not as regular or as frequent as they used to be, then just know that this is normal and you are not necessarily constipated. The volume ejected during bowel movement will decrease as the body absorbs meats efficiently with very little waste.

Summary

You need to keep in mind that digestion issues are real and can occur. When they do, you should be prepared to know the right steps to follow. You should supplement your diet as well. Some of the recommended supplements include Betain HCL with Pepsin, ox bile and Lipase. Also remove any rendered fats or at least limit them in your meals.

Prepare for Social Situations

You should prepare yourself for any eventuality but especially for social situations. It is easy to say anything to people you interact with on a regular basis. For instance, you can go on and on about how you eat junk foods and unhealthy meals all day long and they will probably be fine with it.

But the moment you mention that your meals contain no vegetable, no fruit, and essentially no plant-based fruit, they will think you've gone crazy. This is because most people are accustomed to believing that plant-based are essential or else you will suffer serious consequences. Just remember that you owe nobody an explanation about your choices and you should stress about justifying your actions.

However, you can explain that you are trying out a new diet and testing for allergies and things like that. You can say that it is an experiment that you decided to take on just to see how you will fair. Most people are okay with the experiment aspect and will not pursue it further.

Dining out

Dining out is pretty easy because just about all restaurants and eateries have meat on their menus save for vegan ones. You can ask for a burger or steak patty without anything else. Most restaurants and eateries are very understanding, accommodating with fairly-priced meals.

Obtain Sufficient Sleep

Make sure that you get sufficient amounts of sleep each night. You need to get between seven and nine hours of sleep most nights. If you get good sleep regularly, then all other things in your life will get better. At the onset of the carnivore diet, you are likely to experience some level of insomnia. However, this is a phase that will eventually pass. You should learn a couple of hacks that will enable you to sleep better. Here is a look at some of these hacks.

Work out regularly

Exercising is not only therapeutic but also detoxifies your body. It helps the body to expel toxins. Therefore, if you are receiving wonderful nutrition from all the great food you eat, you should give the body a chance to expel toxins. Sweating expels toxins so make sure that you remain fit and active as you follow the carnivore diet. Regular physical activity is a major part of this lifestyle.

Snacking

You should generally not feel the need to take snacks regularly if you eat enough fatty meat at meal times. The rule is, if you continually feel hungry, then you should eat more meat and also eat fattier cuts. A lot of people have made snacking a habit and may not want to stop immediately. People actually snack even when they are not hungry.

If you really must have a snack, then have pork rinds and similar meats. Make sure that they are not fried or prepared in vegetable oil. According to experience, though, snacking tends to disappear over time. So you can expect your need to have a regular snack fade eventually.

The Carnivore Cleanse

The carnivore cleanse is a revolutionary new way of living where you cleanse your systems, detoxify the body and heal through diet. It is a natural way of eating that supports detoxification and body cleansing.

You will allow the body a much-needed break from all processed, unnatural foods, junk food, as well as grains and carbs. Your body will heal immensely and after a period of time, your health will improve. You will become healthier and will feel like a million dollars.

Chapter Four

The Three Levels of the Carnivore Diet

The carnivore diet is actually a very simple diet. In fact, it is too simple with an equally simple equation that sums it up perfectly.

Carnivore Diet = Meat + Water

Yet this simple equation evokes a lot of questions. There are lots of people wondering whether this diet is sufficient for all their nutrition needs. Ideally, you should start very slowly and progress steadily with time your body learns to tolerate this diet.

Remember to eat as often as possible and to eat till full. However, it will be totally up to you to decide whether to have three, two, or a single meal per day.

The Different Levels of Carnivore Diet

The carnivore diet is best viewed at three different levels. These levels do not aim to make this diet a complex one but simply provide you with a framework that makes it easier for you regardless of your situation. These different levels are level 1, level 2, and level 3.

Level 2 and level 3 are ideally designed to assist you to find the intolerances and sensitive issues that are present due to a diet that causes chronic inflammation. These two levels help you to purify the diet in a way that enables you to then add other foods. These are foods that probably give you more energy, a clear head, excellent health and so on.

As an example, you could be allergic to pork but totally unaware of it. However, this fact could be discovered and eliminated at levels 2 or 3. A lot of dieters thrive at the first level or level 1. It is advisable that you take a few weeks at each level to enable you to determine which foods suit you best and what diseases or adverse symptoms persist.

Level 1 Protocol

At level 1, your diet should consist generally of meat. Anything that is meat or fish or a product of either qualifies to be at this level. There are some exceptions here and these include tea and coffee as well as eggs, butter, whipping cream and cheese.

You can add some dietary supplements at this level. The most suitable supplements during the adaptation stage are electrolytes, pink Himalayan salt, and others such as ox bile, Lipase or Betaine HCL.

You should ensure that you stick with your standard carnivore protocol until you have truly adapted to the diet.

Level 2 Protocol

At level 2, things will be a little bit different. You will have to strictly eat natural meat and meat products only. For instance, you cannot have any processed meats. These are not goo for you because they contain preservatives, additives, and possibly coloring. Avoid processed meats as much as possible.

You should also avoid exceptions and non-meat side snacks. This means you cannot have side dishes like whipping cream, cheese, butter, eggs, coffee or tea. You may also not supplement your diet. At this stage, you are trying to eliminate all these additional foods to observe your body's reaction.

There are some exceptions though because you are allowed to supplement with pink Himalayan salt. You are also allowed some supplements if you are starting at level 2 while skipping level 1.

Level 3 Protocol

At this level, your body will have been used to the diet and will be ready to refine it. This is why you will be expected to consume only grass feed beef and water.
Therefore, expect to feed only on beef and drink only water.

This level is also known as the ultimate carnivore diet and it will help you eliminate all other products, specifically meats that your body may be sensitive to. There are people that are sensitive to pork others are sensitive to certain types of fish and sea foods, and so on. When you consume only high quality beef, then you will easily be able to learn which animals are good for you and which ones are not. You will also be able to track all intolerances you may have and why they occurred.

In brief, at this final level, you should eliminate all other meats and meat products and only have grass fed and grass finished beef. You should also drink water only. Cut out the dairy products, the processed meats, and all others. Eating grass fed meat only is not cheap and will cost you plenty of money. However, it is well worth it.

Beyond the three different levels, you will be in excellent position to perfect and personalize your own diet. You can ideally now begin to look back and see which foods are problematic and which ones are excellent for you. Simply evaluate the foods and how you feel when you eat each. Here is the process;

1. First add regular beef back to your diet (non-grass fed)
2. Next step is to test other meats and see how your body reacts
3. Now try out some eggs and observe your body's reaction
4. Give dairy a try
5. Finally, try both coffee and tea and note your body's reaction

Once you complete the third level for instance, you may choose to add lamb chops or chicken to your diet. When you eventually do, you should also be on the lookout for any symptoms, discomfort and so on.

For instance, let us say you add pork and notice that you feel bloated. In such a case, you should cut it out. Stop eating any product that probably makes you feel any kind of discomfort. If there is any particular meat or meat product that makes you feel great, then you should definitely keep it.

The aim here is to personalize your diet and eating plan to suit your body. Your baseline for the test will be grass fed and finished beef. If you try a eat product and it is okay then you should be free to keep it.

Where to Begin

Ideally, you should start at level 1. This level is the best for all beginners even if you were already on the ketogenic diet. The keto diet is thought to be very close to the carnivore diet.

Sometimes it is advisable for anyone who is not a coffee drinker to begin the carnivore diet at level 2. The reason for this is that it offers the necessary flexibility but without the challenges encountered by those originally on no diet or standard American diet. You should endeavor to spend at least one entire month at a given level before advancing. For instance, if you start at level 1, you should spend at least 30 days at this level before advancing to level 2 and spending a further thirty days here.

Beyond Level 3

Once dieters complete the third level, they usually choose to settle at level one. Majority opt for level 1 while others prefer level 2. Level 1 is less restrictive and accommodates plenty of other products besides grass fed beef. It is crucial that you always remember the baseline for this diet is grass fed as well as finished beef. If you managed to get to level 3 and complete thirty days here, then you will easily be able to determine at which level you belong.

You need to keep in mind that while most people will have settled into the diet after initial metabolic challenges, others may take months to settle down. It is advisable to test for longer just so as to gauge how great the diet is for you and what adjustments you will need to make.

Surviving to the end of level 3 after starting at level one is not an easy feat so congratulations is you manage it. Lots of people sometimes cheat while others are unable to complete all three levels. However, if you know what you want and have your priorities right, then you should be successful eventually.

How to Survive the First Month

The carnivore diet demands that you eat meat and animal products for every meal each day. This amounts to plenty of fat, lots of protein and no carbs. The challenge with this approach is that the body is accustomed to believe grains, fiber, and vegetables are essential nutrients. If this were the case, then conventional wisdom would imply that carnivore dieters experience excessive weight gain, digestive problems, high cholesterol, and other problems.

Fortunately, conventional wisdom is not always accurate. If you closely examine the carnivore diet, you will notice that it is very similar to what our ancestors ate. Many centuries ago, our ancestors ate plenty of meat because it did not make sense to them to gather plenty of vegetables and fruits. Because of this, our bodies became seriously accustomed to a meat-oriented diet.

Historical Observation by Dr. George Ede MD

The world is yet to produce any civilization that ate a vegetarian diet from birth to death. However, there are numerous examples in history of people from varied ethnic, cultural, and geographical backgrounds who ate mostly meat diets for numerous years, lifetimes, and across generations.

Interesting Facts about the Carnivore Diet

Plenty of people love meat and other fatty foods. A diet consisting mostly of meaty foods is easy for most people to consider. Your body goes into ketosis when you eat very little or no carbs at all. Ketosis has been associated with plenty of benefits such as strength gain, weight loss, and mental health challenges like ADHD.

One of the things that you need to avoid is take certain foods even in moderation. For instance, if you eat anything containing sugar or starch, then you may want more. A little sugar is likely to make you desire more. The best solution is to not touch sugar at all. While you may experience some withdrawal symptoms at first, these will subside significantly in due course of time.

On other diets, some cravings might occur and dieters are allowed to cheat occasionally. However, with the carnivore diet, all cravings will very likely disappear and you will not need to have a cheat meal. You will eventually be able to eat your meals without the desire to have other foods, especially junk foods.

Losing weight following the carnivore diet is not just possible but actually comes easy. By religiously pursuing this eating lifestyle, you will drop the pounds and develop strong yet lean muscle.

Challenges and how to overcome them

It is advisable to be aware of the kind of challenges to expect when starting the carnivore diet. Most of these may have been discussed in a different chapter. However, here are a couple of things that you need to be keen on.

You should first go and get your blood tested. You will need to then go back and get tested a second time after about three months. This way, you will be able to note and measure the effects of the diet. You may also want to speak to your doctor or a nutritionist before trying out anything.

Once you begin trying out this diet, you should take note of any changes in your weight, digestive system, and energy levels. Each individual is different and people are affected differently by food and diet. Most people who've tried the carnivore diet have benefited immensely from it. Even then, you should still maintain contact with a healthcare practitioner just so that you stay safe.

Initial week

The first week will most likely also be your toughest. At this stage, you can expect to experience fluctuations in your energy levels, appetite and even focus. To ease this transition, start your journey at a time when you are not too busy but in great overall health. Make sure that you can operate from home, at least for the initial week, or take time off your regular schedule. If you must, ensure that you give yourself sufficient time to sleep.

It is possible to experience certain unexpected challenges. For instance, someone lost appetite for beef yet it is the main ingredient of the carnivore diet. There are numerous reasons that could cause this. However, you should try other options such as lamb chops, chicken, and so on. You can store alternatives like cheese that will help you when you need to snack.

Sometimes the need to cheat during the first week arises. You should try as hard as possible to stay clean and not cheat at all. However, if you really have to cheat, then do so with foods that are not too far from the carnivore diet. For instance, you can have some peanut butter or hazel nuts. While they are not a part of the diet, they are close to it. Compare this to something far out like a rich cream cake.

Appetite swings

You should prepare yourself for occasional appetite swings. On some days you will be able to go several hours without eating. On other days, you may feel hungry just a few hours after a major meal. It is likely though that your appetite will level out after the first couple of weeks so try and hang in there till then. In that time, you will probably have figured out portion sizes for your meals. You should ensure that you have access to quality carnivore food all day everyday.

Some Frequently Asked Questions

Everybody has plenty of questions to ask about this diet especially if they are very new to it. You probably have lots of questions of your own as well. This is common and you should not be afraid to ask questions. Here are some common questions about the carnivore diet.

1. *Are vegetables are allowed with this diet?*

The answer is a distinct no. While you may have all along thought that vegetables are crucial to good health, they may not be that important. Vegetables are a good source of minerals and vitamins but they may not be the best. They tend to contain anti-nutrients which prevent uptake of the nutrients by the body. Veggie nutrients are also largely destroyed by cooking.

2. How do you manage without fiber?

According to experts, if you do not eat plenty of junk food and processed foods, then you will probably not need that much fiber. Basically, fiber is helpful but in this instance where your food is natural, it may not be that necessary.

3. Are you not worried about cholesterol levels?

There is ongoing debate in academic circles as to whether animal fat and meat cause high cholesterol. Cholesterol is affected by plenty of variables. These tend to have a profound effect on your body. There is a huge difference if you take a lot of fat and sugar compared to eating a high fat diet with no sugar. This means that it is the sugar that is the source of the problem and not the fat.

4. Isn't red meat harmful to your body?

There are often plenty of variables at play in life. If you consume plenty of sugary foods and red meat but don't exercise, then your health will definitely be affected. However, if you eat red meat, avoid sugar completely, and workout regularly, then you will be in excellent shape.

5. Should I expect to experience any digestive problems?

It is normal to expect digestive problems with any diet that excludes vegetables. With the carnivore diet, you can expect to only encounter minor discomforts which are quit insignificant compared to other diets. And most of these discomforts will disappear on their own and will generally only be a nuisance than a real cause for concern.

6. Will I need to supplement with micronutrients?

Supplementing with micronutrients is not really necessary especially for the first couple of weeks and months. The aim during the initial stages is to find out how the diet affects micronutrients especially during the first few weeks. Therefore dietary supplements should really be out of question. If you supplement, then you will never get to learn about the deficiencies, if any, or major benefits of this diet.

7. Are organ meats allowed?

Yes, of course. Organ meats should constitute part of your diet. Not only are they highly nutritious but are also very tasty. They provide you with an extra shield of nutrients which your body desperately needs. Organ meats can also be viewed as insurance against any potential nutritional deficiencies.

8. How about the kidneys and all that protein?

There is a myth in the world of nutrition that kidneys and proteins do not get along. It is also a part of the misinformation that tends to discourage dieters from partaking of this diet. There is basically no truth that proteins will adversely affect your kidneys.

9. *Is this diet more or less expensive compared to the standard diet?*

Most people think that costs of both diets are more or less the same. The standard American diet may be cheaper in some instances but costs do not vary that much. Even then, high quality meats and fats are quite costly. Grass-fed cattle and wild caught meat is more expensive compared to grain-fed animals.

<u>Chapter Five</u>

Best Meals for the Carnivore Diet

All-meat or carnivore diet is growing in popularity. Plenty of well-known celebrities and non-celebrities alike are pursuing this diet in one form or another. One of them is Mikhaila Peterson who is the daughter of Jordan B. Peterson. She's on a carnivore diet to ward of an autoimmune disease that almost killed her as a child. Here is a look at some great carnivore meals that you can have any time of day or night.

Breakfast Carnivore Meals

1. California grilled chicken

Ingredients

- o Freshly ground black pepper
- o Kosher salt
- o 1 tsp garlic powder
- o Italian seasoning
- o 4 pieces of skinless, boneless, chicken breasts

Directions

Take a small bowl and mix together garlic powder with Italian seasoning, oil, salt and pepper. Pour this mixture over the chicken and let it marinate for 20 to 30 minutes.

Pre-heat the grill and add the seasoned and marinated chicken breasts. Grill the pieces until properly charred and cooked through. It should take 8 minutes to properly cook each side.

2. Philly Steaks

Ingredients

- o   1 lb thinly sliced flank steak
- o   2 cloves of garlic, diced
- o   Kosher salt
- o   Freshly ground black pepper
- o   Freshly chopped parsley
- o   2 tbsp Italian seasoning
- o   2 tbsp animal oil

Directions

Heat the grill to medium heat. Take a large bowl and mix together the garlic, steak, pepper, animal oil, and season with salt and black pepper. Now place the mixture in foil packs.

Fold up the packs nicely and put them in the grill. Grill the steak for about 10 minutes. It should be nicely cooked now. Allow to cook for a further two minutes. Garnish with parsley and serve.

3. Scrambled Eggs and Milk

Ingredients

- o   A pinch of salt
- o   Freshly ground black pepper
- o   Some animal fat/oil
- o   2 medium-size eggs
- o   1 glass of milk

Preparation

Heat a shallow pan or skillet over medium heat on a stove. Pour in some of the fat and let it heat for a minute. Take the eggs and break over the pan or skillet. Use a wooden or plastic spoon to prevent the egg from sticking onto the pan.

Place the egg onto a plate and season with the salt and pepper. Now warm the milk in a sauce pan and then pour it into a glass.

4. Pork Shoulder Cutlets

Ingredients
- 1.5 pounds of boneless pork shoulder divided into 4 parts
- 2 large eggs
- ¾ cup animal oil
- Sea salt
- Freshly ground pepper

Preparation

Take the pork steaks and pound between double layer plastic wrap. Take a bowl and lightly beat the eggs. Add some cornstarch and season with the freshly ground black pepper as well as the kosher salt.

Take the cutlets and season individually with pepper and kosher salt. Transfer to the egg mixture and coat them generously. Take a skillet and put on the stove at medium heat. Heat some of the oil and cook the cutlets two at a time. Allow them to cook for three minutes at a time. You may now remove them from the heat and place on a wire rack then season with pepper and salt.

6. Pan Ranch Pork Chops

Ingredients

- o   4 pieces of 8-ounce pork chops
- o   2 tbsp of oil
- o   Packaged ranch seasoning
- o   3 cloves of sliced and diced garlic
- o   Freshly ground black pepper
- o   Kosher salt

Directions

First pre-heat the oven till 400 degrees F. Take a baking sheet, oil it lightly and then place the pork chops on it. Pour some more oil and add the salt and pepper to taste. Take the Ranch Seasoning and add to the pork chops.

Place the baking sheet with the seasoned pork chops into the oven. Let them cook for a while until well and thoroughly cooked. They will get to an internal temperature of about 140 degrees F when properly cooked. Now broil for about two to three minutes until the meat turns a nice brown color or becomes slightly charred. The meat is now ready to serve. The cooking time for this particular meal will depend on the thickness or size of the pork chops.

7. Baked Chicken Fingers

Ingredients

- o   1 pound of skinless, boneless chicken cutlets
- o   Kosher salt
- o   Freshly ground black pepper
- o   2 large, beaten eggs
- o   3 tbsp animal oil

Directions

First pre-heat the oven to a temperature of 425 degrees F then take a baking sheet and line it with foil. Take the chicken cutlets and cut them into strips of about one and a half inches. Season the cutlets with salt and pepper.

Dip the chicken strips in the eggs and then transfer the strips to the baking sheet. Now, once all the chicken strips are on the baking sheet, let them cook in the hot oven for 10 to 12 minutes or until they turn golden brown. Now heat broiler until it turns a nice golden brown.

Your chicken is now ready so remove from the oven, place on a plate carefully and serve whilst still nice and hot. Enjoy the chicken fillets.

8. Fish Fingers

Ingredients

- o   2.5 pounds fish fillet
- o   2 beaten eggs
- o   ½ tsp of garlic powder
- o   Kosher salt
- o   Freshly ground black pepper
- o   2 tbsp Animal fat

Directions

Take a deep frying pan and pre-heat the oil. Slice the fish into long, thin, strips.
Combine the garlic powder with some salt, and pepper in a bowl. Beat the eggs thoroughly in another bowl.

Now dip the fish fingers in the salt, and pepper mixture. Make sure that they are evenly coated. Put the fish fingers in the pan and fry till golden brown or for about 2 to 3 minutes. Remove from the pan and place on a plate. Serve while hot.

9. Grilled lamb chops

Ingredients

- o   2 tbsp garlic powder
- o   A pinch of cayenne powder
- o   Sea salt
- o   2 tbsp animal fat/oil
- o   6 lamb chops about ½-inch thick

Procedure

Use a food processor and add the assorted spices then combine them so they mix properly. Add the animal fat and mix further. Take the paste and apply it onto the lamb chops. Allow them to marinade for about an hour.

Take a grill pan and place it on the stove at high heat. Add the chops and let the sear for 2 to 3 minutes. Now turn them over and sear some more for another 2 to 3 minutes. They should be cooked now so place them on a plate and serve while hot.

10. Chicken Wings

Ingredients

- o   12 pieces of chicken wings rinsed and dried
- o   2 tbsp animal fat/oil
- o   1 tbsp toasted sesame seeds
- o   Freshly ground black pepper
- o   Kosher salt
- o   Franks RedHot sauce

Preparation

Pre-heat your oven to a temperature of 400 degrees F.
Take the chicken wings and season them adequately with the salt and pepper. Pour a little oil on them and let them sit for a couple of minutes.

Take a baking sheet and lay the wings. Put the sheet in the oven and bake for about half an hour or until the wings turn a nice brown color and are cooked through.

Prepare your meat only sauce and simmer on low heat. Enjoy the chicken wings with the sauce while still hot.

Carnivore Lunch Meals

1. Grilled Buffalo Wings

Ingredients

- o 1 tsp freshly ground black pepper
- o 1 tsp of garlic powder
- o 3 lbs whole chicken wings
- o 1 tsp kosher salt
- o 1/3 cup of hot sauce

Directions

Take a small bowl and combine the pepper, salt and garlic powder. Take a large bowl and put the wings then add the seasoning mixture of salt, garlic, and pepper. Make sure the chicken wings are evenly coated.

Pre-heat a grill oven to a temperature of 350 degrees F. Take the wings and place them in the grill. Make sure that they are closely touching each other. This is the complete opposite of conventional grilling where space between the pieces is necessary to prevent steaming.

In this case, steaming is necessary to keep them moist. Flip the wings occasionally and grill for about 20 minutes. Take a shallow pan and heat the sauce on low heat. Whisk the mixture so the ingredients mix thoroughly.

Take the wings out of the oven toss them in the sauce ensuring they are generously coated and place back in the oven. Allow them to sit in the oven for an additional 2 minutes then serve while hot.

2. Grilled Strip Steaks

Ingredients

- o   1 tsp dried garlic powder
- o   3 strip steaks 1.5 inches thick
- o   1 tsp chipotle Chile powder
- o   1.5 tbsp animal fat
- o   1 tsp red pepper flakes
- o   Freshly ground black pepper
- o   Kosher salt

Directions

Take a small bowl and combine the black pepper with the kosher salt, chipotle powder, garlic and red pepper flakes. Mix the ingredients thoroughly and then let it sit.

Take the steaks and pat them dry using paper towels. Then place the steaks in a mid-sized baking dish. Rub the steaks with some oil and then pour some seasoning generously on them. Make sure that all the pieces are generously covered with the seasoning mix.

Now cover the bowl and let it sit for about an hour or two so that the flavors can penetrate the steaks. Once the steak pieces are properly marinated, heat the grill and place the steaks on a tray. Place the tray in the grill and let the steaks cook for a couple of minutes. Turn each side after two minutes and then turn again so that all sides are cooked.

Once the steaks are nicely cooked, transfer them to a plate and cover them tightly using aluminum foil. Let the steaks rest for a couple of minutes. Now remove the foil after a quarter of an hour. If not then the steaks will continue to cook. Take a large knife and slice the steaks. Check if the salt is sufficient and sprinkle some more if necessary. Serve while hot.

3. Chicken Cutlets

Ingredients

- o   2 large eggs
- o   4 pieces of boneless, skinless, chicken cutlets
- o   2 tbsp Animal oil
- o   1 tbsp Mustard powder
- o   Freshly ground black pepper
- o   Kosher salt

Preparation

Take a shallow bowl and beat the eggs.. Season the mixture with both salt and pepper. Take the chicken pieces and season with the kosher salt and black pepper.

Put the chicken pieces in the bowl with the beaten eggs and ensure they are well coated. Remove from the egg bowl and add the ,mustard seed.

Heat the oil in a large skillet over medium-heat. Cook the cutlets and add some more oil. Let it cook for about 4 minutes. Once cooked, place the chicken pieces on paper towel-lined plate.

4. Monster Meat Balls

Ingredients
- o   1 cup of milk
- o   ½ pounds of ground turkey
- o   2 tbsp of garlic powder
- o   ¼ cup parsley for garnish
- o   1 large diced and sliced onion
- o   Parsley
- o   2 tbsp animal oil

Preparation

Take the turkey and place it in a bowl. Add, garlic, parsley, pepper and some salt. Pour in some milk and mix together. Add some bread crumbs to help bind the ingredients and form meat balls. Now form three or four oversized meatballs.

Turn on the oven and heat some oil on medium heat. Take the meatballs whilst still in the small pot and place them in the oven. Let them sear over the surface for a while and keep moving them around. This helps to maintain their round shape.

Now remove the meatballs from the oven and add the sauce and some water. Ensure that they are covered completely by the sauce and place back in the oven. Let is sit for a while and allow it to simmer. Cover the sauce pan as the turkey meatballs simmers and ensure to keep turning them occasionally.

5. Beef Stew

Ingredients

- o   2 tbsp oil
- o   2.5 pounds of beef chuck sliced into 2-inch cubes
- o   Freshly ground black pepper
- o   Kosher salt
- o   2 tbsp garlic powder
- o   Fresh spices
- o   10 cups of beef or chicken broth or water

Directions

Heat the large Dutch oven over medium heat. Generously pour some animal oil in the pan and fill it about ¼ of the way up. Use the salt and pepper to season the beef pieces and then add them to the pan. Now sauté some of the beef pieces and stir occasionally. Keep going until the pieces turn a nice brown color. This will probably take about 8 minutes.

Now sauté the rest of the beef pieces and a further 8 minutes later transfer the beef from the pan to a plate.

6. BBQ Chicken Drumsticks

Ingredients

- o   1 teaspoon of paprika
- o   Freshly ground black pepper
- o   Kosher salt
- o   12 pieces of chicken drumsticks
- o   2 tbsp garlic powder
- o   ½ a cup of water
- o   Some oil or animal fat

Directions

Take a small bowl and mix together the paprika, salt, black pepper, and any other seasoning. Use this spicy mixture to season the drumsticks. Make sure that you loosen the skin before seasoning the meat. Once you have nicely and generously seasoned all the drumsticks, cover them carefully using plastic wrap then let them marinate overnight or for at least an hour.

Get the grill ready and pre-heat to medium heat. Use the oil on the grill grate to prevent the chicken drums from sticking. Proceed to grill the chicken and keep turning it until it is properly and thoroughly cooked. Check that the skin is crisp. This should take about 25 or so minutes. Remove from the grill once ready and place them on a plate. Serve the drumsticks while still hot.

7. Mexican Fish Stew

Ingredients

- o   4 tilapia fish fillets, each cut into 4 pieces
- o   Freshly ground pepper and kosher salt
- o   2 tbsp animal fat/oil
- o   2 tbsp ground garlic powder
- o   1 tbsp chili powder

Directions

Take a shallow dish and put in the fish fillet pieces. Get the seasoning and season the fish generously. This includes the salt, pepper, and garlic powder. Now take a large skillet and put it on the stove on medium heat. Add some oil and seasoning then put the fish to the skillet.

Get some hot water or broth and add to the fish. Let it cook and stir slightly until cooked. Check for seasoning and add some more salt or pepper if necessary. Your Mexican fish stew is now ready to serve. Serve while hot.

8. Marinated Chicken Breasts

Ingredients

- o   3 tsp dried herbs
- o   2 tbsp vinegar
- o   2 tsp garlic powder
- o   Freshly ground pepper and kosher salt
- o   4 pieces of skinless, boneless chicken breasts
- o   ¼ cup of oil

Directions

Take the vinegar and assorted herbs and powders and pour them into a sealable plastic bag. Add some oil to the mixture then shake the bag and all its ingredients. Ensure that the ingredients mix thoroughly.

Now open the bag and place the chicken breast pieces inside. Shut the bag and shake it thoroughly so that the oil and seasoning mixture coats the chicken pieces evenly. You can freeze these for a while if you like.

Remove the plastic bag from the freezer, thaw in the microwave, then place on a pan. Heat a grill pan or grill and when it turns hot place the chicken breast pieces. Let the chicken cook for at least 4 minutes then turn sides and cook for a further 4 minutes. Ensure that the pieces are properly cooked. The chicken is now ready to serve.

9. Oven Roasted Lamb Shanks

Ingredients

- o   3 tbsp animal oil
- o   Freshly ground black pepper and kosher salt
- o   4 pieces of lamb shanks
- o   4 tbsp mixed herbs
- o   3 cups of water

Directions

Preheat the oven then heat the animal oil over high heat in a medium Dutch oven until the oil starts to smoke. Take the shanks and pour the mixed herbs seasoning on both sides. Add to the heat and let them sear until they turn into a beautiful golden brown color on both sides.

Once the golden brown beautiful color is observed, the shanks are ready and can be removed and placed onto a plate. Prepare a soup, broth, or sauce and then enjoy the lamb shanks with the broth.

10. Mexican Chicken Soup

Ingredients

- o   2 whole or 4 split chicken breasts with skin and bone
- o   Some animal oil
- o   3 tbsp garlic powder
- o   2 tbsp mixed dry herbs
- o   1 tsp ground cumin
- o   1 tsp coriander seed

Instructions

Preheat your oven at a temperature of 350 degrees F. Take a sheet pan then place the chicken breasts on it. Pour some oil then sprinkle some pepper and salt. Roast the chicken breasts for about 40 minutes. Once cooked let it sit for a while then remove the bones and skin.

Shred the meat then cover it and put it aside. Now you can prepare your favorite broth or warm some if you have. Put the broth in a saucepan, place on the stove on medium heat then add the chicken pieces. Season the mixture to taste using the mixed herbs then add some more salt and pepper if necessary.

Let the soup boil and then lower the heat. Let it simmer for about 5 to 7 minutes before removing from the heat. Your chicken soup is now ready to serve. You should serve it hot and enjoy this delicious meal.

Dinner Carnivore Meals

1. Hawaiian Roasted Pork

Ingredients

- o   2 tbsp freshly ground black pepper
- o   3 tbsp coarse or Hawaiian salt
- o   2 pieces of boneless pork rump roasts
- o   2 tbsp of oil
- o   Natural herbs

½ cup of water
1 tbsp mixed natural herbs

Instructions

Place the pork roasts on a plate and season them with the pepper and salt. Prepare an outdoor barbecue using wood chips soaked in water and add to the coals.

Place the pork on the hot grill and sear in order to lock in all the natural juices. Season the pork with the natural herbs. Roast the pork for a further 3 hours and cover the grill. It should now be ready to serve so shred the meat using two forks.

2. Pan Fried Tilapia

Ingredients

- o   ½ tsp fresh ground black pepper
- o   1 teaspoon sea salt
- o   1.5 pounds of fresh tilapia fish fillets
- o   2 tsp mixed seasoning
- o   2 tbsp butter
- o   1 tsp ground garlic

Instructions

Preheat the oven to about 300 degrees F. Take a shallow baking dish and thoroughly mix the seasoning with pepper, salt. Place the tilapia fillets in the seasoning and coat both sides generously. Shake off any excess then place the fish in a skillet.

Sear the fish on both sides for about 2 minutes each side. Once both sides turn a nice brown color, remove from the skillet and transfer to a baking sheet lined with paper towels or a paper grocery bag. Put the fish in the oven to maintain the warmth.

Turn down the heat to low and then add the butter. Let the butter melt all over the fish in order to add flavor. Add more of the natural herbs and allow to sauté for about 2 minutes. Remove the fish and place on a platter or serving plates.

3. Grilled Prime Ribs

Ingredients

- o   2 tbsp garlic powder
- o   Freshly ground black pepper
- o   3 prime rib-eye steaks
- o   Mixture of dried seasoning
- o   Some animal based cooking oil

Instructions

Preheat the grill to 350 degrees F. Take the steaks and season them generously in a bowl. Ensure that both sides are seasoned with the salt, pepper, and the seasoning. After the seasoning, set aside and let it sit.

Form a paste using the garlic and set it aside. Now take a small skillet and place it on the stove over medium heat and add some oil. Once the oil starts heating up, add the garlic paste and stir thoroughly. Now allow the oil to come to a boil then let it simmer for a while. Add some seasoning and then cook until it turns a nice golden brown color.

Remove the skillet from the heat and let the garlic cool still in the oil. Mix it some more till it becomes a paste. Now put the meat on top of a hot grill then cook till it turns a nice brown color on both sides. It should take about 5 minutes for one side and 3 minutes for the other side.

Take the garlic paste and smear over the meat. Make sure that the steaks are facing upwards and place on the grill rack in the stove. Cook some more for about 10 minutes for rare. Remove from the grill and let it sit for about 10 minutes. Transfer the meat from the grill onto a chopping board then proceed to cut the meat between the bone and flesh of each steak. It is now ready to serve.

4. Perfect Roast Turkey

Ingredients

- o   1 tbsp assorted dry spices
- o   ¼ lbs of unsalted butter
- o   1 large, fresh turkey weighing 15 – 20 lbs
- o   Freshly ground pepper and kosher salt
- o   2 tbsp Dried garlic and onion

Procedure

First pre-heat the oven to a temperature of 350 degrees F. Now melt the butter in a small pan and add the seasoning. Set this mixture aside. Take the turkey and wash it thoroughly after removing the giblets. Remove any leftover feathers if present then dry the outside by patting.

Take a large roasting pan and place the turkey in it. Pour some salt and pepper on the inside of the turkey cavity. Now pour some seasoning on the inside as well. Take the butter mixture and brush the turkey on the outside. Now tie the turkey legs together using tuck and string beneath the bird.

Roast the turkey in the grill for about 3 hours or until the juices run clear if you cut the turkey between the thigh and the leg. Take the turkey from the grill and place it on a cutting board. Ensure that you cover it with aluminum foil to maintain the heat and juices. Let the bird rest for about 20 to 30 minutes. Find some large sharp knives then slice the turkey the right way. It is now ready to serve.

5. Goat meat Stew

Ingredients

- o 2 tbsp oil
- o 2.5 pounds of goat meat chuck sliced into 2-inch cubes
- o Freshly ground black pepper
- o Coarse kosher salt
- o 2 tbsp garlic powder
- o Fresh spices
- o 10 cups of goat or chicken broth or water

Directions

Heat a large Dutch oven over medium heat. Generously pour some animal fat or oil in the pan and fill it about ¼ of the way up. Use the salt and pepper to season the beef pieces and then add them to the pan.

Now sauté some of the goat meat pieces and stir occasionally. Keep going until the pieces turn a nice brown color. This will probably take about 8 minutes. Now sauté the rest of the meat pieces and a further 8 minutes later transfer the beef from the pan to a plate.

6. Pan-fried Beef Liver

Ingredients

- o   1 tbsp ground garlic
- o   2 tbsp freshly ground black pepper
- o   2 tbsp coarse sea salt
- o   1 large beef liver, cut up into small cubic chunks
- o   1 cup dried mixed herbs
- o   ¼ cup animal oil

Procedure

Place the beef liver pieces in a bowl. Add salt and pepper then pour in the seasoning. Mix it thoroughly then set it aside for about 15 minutes. Take a skillet and put it on the stove at medium heat. Add the oil and heat if for about a minute.

Now pour in the liver and all the seasoning. Reduce the heat to low and let it cook for about 10 minutes. Cover the skillet so as to hold in the flavors. Check it occasionally and add some water. Pour in the garlic powder then cover and leave for 2 to 3 more minutes.

Take the skillet off the heat and set it aside. The liver should be cooked and should have a nice, thick stew. Taste and add some salt or pepper if necessary. Your beef liver is now ready to serve.

7. Bacon and Cheese Omelet

Ingredients

- o   Freshly ground black pepper
- o   ¼ cup parmesan cheese
- o   1 tsp ground garlic
- o   2 large eggs
- o   Coarse sea salt
- o   3 slices of bacon
- o   1 tbsp animal oil

Instructions

Cut up the bacon into thin strips. Season the bacon strips and set aside. Chop up the parmesan cheese. Set aside as well. Take a pan and put it on the stove on low heat. Pour some oil on the pan.

Take a small bowl and beat the eggs. Add salt and pepper to taste. Pour the beaten eggs onto the pan and spread out. Add the bacon onto the eggs and let it cook for just a couple of seconds. Now pour in the parmesan cheese together with the dried garlic.

Turn the omelet and allow the other side to cook. This should cook for about 1 minute and the omelet is ready. The bacon strips should turn a nice brown color. Check for salt and sprinkle some more if necessary. Place the omelet on a plate and you are now ready to serve.

8. Grilled Tuna Steaks

Ingredients

- o   2 tbsp fish or animal oil
- o   Freshly ground black pepper
- o   Coarse sea salt
- o   1 tbsp freshly ground and dried garlic
- o   4 fresh tuna steaks, each 1 inch thick

Procedure

First turn on the grill to a high heat. Take the tune fish steaks and brush on the oil. Turn the steaks around and brush some more oil. Sprinkle each steak with salt and pepper.

Place the tuna fish steaks into the grill and ensure that you grill each side for about 2 ½ minutes only. Make sure to turn the other side once done. Remember to leave the center raw otherwise the tune will become dry and tough. Let the steaks rest for about 5 minutes and serve.

9. Grilled Beef Tenderloin

Ingredients

- o   2 tbsp animal or fish oil
- o   2 tsp coarse sea salt
- o   4 beef fillet pieces, 6 to 8 ounces each
- o   Freshly ground black pepper

Preparation

Take the beef fillet pieces from the refrigerator about a half hour before cooking. Turn on the grill to medium heat. Place the beef fillets in a bowl and apply the oil lightly using a brush. Pour some salt and seasoning on the beef fillets to taste.

Now place them on the grill for a bout 4 minutes without turning until grill marks begin to appear. Turn on the beef fillets and let them cook for a further 4 to 5 minutes. The beef fillets are now ready to serve. You can enjoy the delicious meat with a sauce of choice. Bone broth would be great in this instance or a beef stew.

10. Spicy Chicken Stew

Ingredients

- o   2 tbsp dried freshly ground red pepper
- o   2 tbsp freshly ground black pepper
- o   1 tbsp coriander seeds
- o   1 tbsp cumin seeds
- o   2 tbsp coarse sea salt
- o   Tender chicken cut up into pieces
- o   1 tbsp dried spices
- o   ½ cup warm water

Procedure

Take the chicken pieces and place them in the bowl. Add some spices and seasoning. Let the chicken sit and marinate for about 15 minutes. Put a large saucepan on medium heat on the stove. Pour in the oil and add the chicken pieces.

Turn the heat to low and cover the sauce pan. Let the chicken cook for a couple of minutes. Open the pan and season the chicken with the red pepper, black pepper, and salt. Cover the pan and let the chicken continue to cook. After 10 minutes, open the pan and pour in a little warm water.

Cover the pan and let the stew simmer. Taste the stew and add some salt, seasoning, or pepper to taste. Allow it to simmer for a further five minutes. If the stew is thick enough and sufficiently seasoned, remove from the stove and set aside.

Your chicken stew is now ready to serve. It should have a nice, tasty, thick stew which you can pour into a cup. Enjoy your delicious spicy chicken and the thick stew.

Carnivore Snacks

1. Boiled eggs

Take some eggs and add them to boiling water. Boil the eggs for 3 to 8 minutes depending on how you like them. 3 minutes for soft boiled and 5 to 8 minutes for hard boiled. Remove the shell then add some salt to taste.

2. Chicken nuggets

Simply take some chicken pieces, season with your favorite seasoning and grill for a couple of minutes on medium heat.

3. Sunnyside up egg

You will need an egg and salt. Simply fry an egg using a shallow pan. Just fry one side without breaking the yolk. Season the egg with salt and pepper and then transfer to a plate.

4. Fried chicken entrails

Simply fry chicken entrails on a pan. Add some oil and seasoning. Cook for 3 to 5 minutes only.

5. Left over beef chunks

You can warm some left over beef chunks and have them for a mid-morning or afternoon snack

6. Bacon slices

Season some bacon and fry them on a shallow frying pan on low heat

7. Beef sausages

Boil some beef sausages then season before frying on a shallow skillet

8. Fish fingers

Fish fingers are easy to prepare. You can buy them at the grocery store and simply cook them on a skillet on low heat for a few minutes

9. Meat balls

Meatballs are easy to prepare. Mince your preferred meat and season it then mould into spherical shape. Grill in the oven for 10 - 15 minutes.

10. Prawns

Prepare prawns and season them appropriately. Have them for your evening snack

Chapter Six

Benefits of the Carnivore Diet

Major benefits of the carnivore diet

It reduces inflammation

The carnivore diet has many benefits. It is considered as the lead anti-inflammatory diet for patients suffering autoimmune conditions. It also has numerous other health benefits.

This diet lowers your insulin levels significantly. Anyone suffering from insulin-related challenges like diabetes will benefit from lower insulin levels. Some patients have testified of getting cured of diabetes.

Simple eating method

The carnivore diet provides a simple way of eating. Dieters pursuing this way of eating do not have to count calories or eat at certain times. This diet requires you to eat as much as you can whenever you want. You eat to satisfaction without any concern and will still lose weight.

Some people worry about counting calories, meal preparations, and macronutrients, and so on. ***All these worries are fortunately not valid with the carnivore diet.***

Your digestive system will improve

While there is no fiber associated with the carnivore diet, it does promote a healthy digestive system. There is reason to believe that cutting fiber from your diet actually improves your digestive system.

Improved mental clarity

You will enjoy improved mental clarity just like those on the keto diet do. Our brains are made up of 60% fat so a diet with plenty of fat will support the brain. Experts attribute improved mental clarity to restricted carbs intake with increase protein and fat intake.

Reduced inflammation

According to a 3-month study by health practitioners in the US state of Georgia, it was established that persons on a low carb, high fat diet had lower inflammation levels in general compared to those on a high carb, low fat diet.

Faster weight loss

Despite common presumption, you will actually lose weight faster on the carnivore diet. The body usually accumulates fat because it is not insulin sensitive. This means that any time you consume carbs, they are converted into fat. However, if you completely cut out carbs from your diet, your body will become extremely sensitive to insulin. Your hunger hormones are regulated so that you do not eat unnecessarily.

Improves testosterone levels

High fat diets have been shown to improve testosterone levels. It is known that testosterone levels tend to decrease with age. This is a situation that can be changed and turned around through the high fat, high protein diet.

It helps improve condition of patients with autoimmune conditions

Plenty of patients with autoimmune conditions like MS have seen their symptoms improve drastically by practicing and following the carnivore diet. It is also great for patients with chronic conditions like high blood pressure and diabetes.

It cleanses and detoxifies the body

By taking the carnivore diet, you will help to cleanse your body and eliminate toxins.

Worthwhile lifestyle to pursue

To many people, the carnivore diet sounds a little crazy. They think it is a highly risky and deficient diet that will harm the body. This is actually not true. There are numerous anecdotal testaments of people who have experienced significant weight loss, increased mental focus, and improved health and mood markers that make it hard to ignore the diet.

A diet that restricts the consumption of unnecessary calories especially from carbs will definitely benefit your body. You will actually lose weight while enjoying a juicy steak and delicious ribs.

Intermittent Fasting and the Carnivore Diet

Intermittent fasting is a lifestyle that requires you to fast for a period of time then have your meals during another much smaller window. You will generally fast for much longer with an eating window of only a few hours.

While the carnivore diet dictates that you eat as much as you can whenever you want, intermittent fasting calls for alternate periods of fasting and eating. However, it is possible to incorporate intermittent fasting with your all-meat diet.

The good news is that it is possible to follow an intermittent fasting lifestyle with the carnivore diet. **This is because meat is very satisfying so you are able to go for lengthy periods of time without eating.**

Intermittent fasting does not dictate the foods that you eat but only provides eating and fasting windows. Therefore, during your eating windows you will strictly adhere to the carnivore diet.

What to Expect with Intermittent Fasting

- o You can expect to lose lots of weight, much more than you would on a normal diet
- o You will not feel hungry regularly as you would on a regular diet
- o Most of your cravings will disappear
- o Your allergies will also disappear with time
- o Expect to have a clear head
- o Your body will be more efficient in cleansing and detoxification

Conclusion

The next step is to begin following this diet as instructed. You can do this slowly- following one step at a time. The best level to begin at is level one. Follow the instructions provided and proceed all the way to level three.

Within a few short weeks or months, you will begin to enjoy the numerous benefits of this diet. Your initial challenges will eventually disappear and you will begin to feel great. You will also be in a great position to heal your body and see all the symptoms of any chronic conditions disappear.

Subscribe to our Carnivore Diet blog at:

www.CarnivoreCleanse.com

References

Health.com
https://www.health.com/nutrition/carnivore-diet

Meat Health
https://meat.health/knowledge-base/carnivore-diet-what-to-eat/

Everyday Health
https://www.everydayhealth.com/diet-nutrition/diet/carnivore-diet-benefits-risks-food-list-more/

ONNIT Academy
https://www.onnit.com/academy/the-carnivore-diet/

<u>Book Three</u>

Apple Cider Vinegar Benefits

"Natural Weight Loss and Health Benefits, Glowing Health and Skin, Natural Cures, and Alkaline Healing with Apple Cider Vinegar"

By Dana Lee

"Twenty years from now you will be more disappointed by the things that you didn't do than by the ones you did do. So throw off the bowlines. Sail away from safe harbor. Catch the trade winds in your sails. Explore. Dream. Discover."

*~ **Mark Twain***

Table of Contents

Introduction

The goal of this book is to positively impact the reader's experience in any way possible, even if just a minuscule amount, be it from a word, sentence, idea or comment in this book; then we have made a positive impact and achieved our goal.

"Apple Cider Vinegar - Is the one of the most under-rated natural health supplements out there – WHY?"

I created this book because I do not like to see so many people being charged high prices for sophisticated health supplements and programs, most of which are not natural. Apple cider vinegar is available in most food stores and has huge life-changing effects on health and appearance. I speak from personal experience.

The science and history for apple cider vinegar's health benefits are tremendous and go back for thousands of years! Compare this fact to some of the modern health supplements being used.

<u>My Quick Personal Story With Apple Cider Vinegar</u>

When I was only 26 years old I was suffering from multiple symptoms of poor nutrition and stress.

- Weight issues
- Spiking blood pressure syndrome
- Weird sensations in my ankles and feet if standing for long periods
- Bad skin and appearance – generally always feeling unhealthy.

At that time, I worked a government job on 3rd shift for over 6 years. I was not healthy at all and was borderline pre-diabetic; I weighed nearly 205 pounds, and was always feeling sick or tired.

After several 'wake-up calls" I eventually started a manageable work-out routine and ran 1-2 miles every other day, which helped me significantly and I lost a lot of weight, but my average blood pressure was still around 160/90 and I still had a high body fat percentage. I wasn't over-weight but I still had a lot of subcutaneous fat, it was very strange and hard to figure out how to get rid of it and lower my BP to a normal range.

When I reached the age of 29, I quit my job to become an entrepreneur and decided to do whatever it also took to really reclaim my health since I was going to need it now. After a few more scares with super high blood pressure episodes and just generally always feeling sick, I discovered one of the first health supplements that would begin the PERMANENT and sustaining health turnaround for me.

I must say, my personal experience with Apple Cider Vinegar for health benefits has been very noticeable, especially when I drink it consistently. All my biomarkers are very strong and I hover around 8-10% body fat. I do not eat any kind of special diet, just <u>clean healthy</u> food, and the apple cider vinegar in morning or before bed, combined with a light work-out routine consisting of 45 minutes 6 days a week..SIMPLE.

Although this was only ONE component of my new healthy lifestyle, it has played a major, if not the best, role in my drastic health and energy improvements. The truth is that I actually <u>feel and look significantly better than I did when I was 29</u>, and I wrote this at age 39.

This book is for someone just starting off in their quest for natural, healthy and beneficial supplementation; Apple Cider Vinegar is definitely something that has worked for a lot of people for a very long time. How can we ignore such a great history of positive results revolving around something so readily available in our stores and so affordable?

Apple cider vinegar has been called a superfluid, capable of doing everything from polishing your furniture to lowering your cholesterol levels. In this book, we will go over some of the anecdotal and scientific benefits of this fluid. Here is some of what apple cider vinegar can do:

Helps Reduce Appetite:

A study done in Sweden in 2005 discovered that people were more satisfied and fuller for longer periods when they ate bread along with vinegar, as opposed to by itself. The great ingredient in vinegar that reduces appetite is thought to be acetic acid.

This substance can help to lower foods' glycemic indexes. In other words, it slows down the rate that sugars get released into your blood stream, reducing your urge to eat more.

Lowers Fat Levels in the Body:

Many people insist that apple cider vinegar can help to shed weight, but there isn't as much scientific evidence for this. One study, done in Japan, however, showed that overweight people who drank acetic acid with water over about three months showed significant weight loss.

Lowers Levels of Bad Cholesterol:
A study done in 2012 by Life Science found that consuming apple cider vinegar over two months could reduce bad blood lipids significantly. These harmful blood lipids add to high levels of cholesterol.

Makes your Hair Shinier:
Apple cider vinegar can be used as a conditioner supplement or replacement. Just add one part apple cider vinegar to an equal amount of water and let it soak on your hair for a few minutes, then rinse thoroughly.

The rinsing step is important unless you want to smell like vinegar! These are just a few examples of what apple cider vinegar can do, but the rest of this book will go into detail about the other wonders this miracle liquid can offer you.

The final chapter will explore a bonus subject, using apple cider vinegar to cure and get rid of cellulite. We will also cover some other natural methods to use along with the vinegar for extra effectiveness in this.

Thank you for Choosing this Book:
There are plenty of books on this subject on the market, thanks again for choosing this one! Every effort was made to ensure it is full of as much useful information as possible. Please enjoy!

Chapter 1: What is Apple Cider Vinegar?

New research has suggested that ingesting apple cider vinegar can fight diabetes, help people lose weight, lower blood pressure levels, and aid acid reflex problems.

The wonderful advantages of apple cider vinegar arise from its amazing compounds that heal, including the acetic acid mentioned in the introduction, along with enzymes, probiotics, magnesium, and potassium.

Raw, organic apple cider vinegar is an effective natural health supplement that can be used each day. You can use this to detox your body, help you digest the food you eat, and to get a fast energy burst that is healthier than coffee.

In addition, you can include apple cider vinegar into your personal care routine to whiten your teeth, make your hair softer, and even to clean your kitchen. Chapter three will cover other beauty benefits of this liquid in greater detail.

Regular vs. Raw Apple Cider Vinegar:

Apple cider vinegar (the unfiltered variety) can be made from water and apple juice, but in this case, it probably isn't pasteurized, and the "mother" has not yet been filtered out. It has a cloudy appearance and might have some sediment in the bottom of the bottle.

Killing the bad, Helping the Good Grow:

The acetic acid present in apple cider vinegar has the capability of killing off dangerous bacteria while also supporting the growth of healthy bacteria. Since this acid kills off dangerous bacteria as soon as it contacts it, it basically functions as a gentle, natural antibiotic for your body.

So apple cider vinegar can provide your body natural benefits in regards to higher immunity to diseases, digestion aid, and nicer skin without side effects. Of course, for some people, there may be exceptions. We will cover side effects and possible interactions later on in the book so you can stay safe.

A Great Source of Polyphenols:

In addition to the benefits already mentioned, apple cider vinegar is a quality source for something called polyphenols. Studies support the fact that polyphenols can help to prevent cancer, diabetes, osteoporosis, cardiovascular issues, and diseases such as Alzheimer's.

Similar to Fermented Liquids:

Just like other fermented products, apple cider vinegar can be made using sugar combined with active yeast. When this happens, people use the naturally occurring source of sugar that crushed apples provide.

The sugar gets consumed by the yeast and uses it to create healthy bacteria, which is the process of fermentation in a nutshell.

Organic Sources:

The absolute best sources of apple cider vinegar for health, therapeutic, and wellness purposes should come from apples that are certified organic. Pasteurization isn't crucial and isn't even recommended if you want to use it for health-related reasons since pasteurization kills off the enzymes and delicate nutrients in the liquid.

The Prevention of Bad Bacteria:

Vinegar's acidity helps to prevent bad bacteria, such as E. Coli for example, from developing. Once the process of fermentation is complete, acetic acid has formed, the major advantageous compound present in apple cider vinegar.

<u>Unattractive Apple Cider Vinegar is a Good Sign:</u>

Some new users may be put off by the fact that apple cider vinegar can look murky and have strings that look like cobwebs inside them. However, this is a great sign!

The brown, murky appearance of apple cider vinegar, along with the yeast strands that you might see, can actually be an indication that the apple cider vinegar is high-quality liquid. The strands are live yeasts that are actually living. These strands have bacteria that will provide amazing health benefits once they enter your body.

Apple Cider Vinegar Hardly Has Sugar or Calories:

Though you make apple cider vinegar with sugar, the fermentation process causes the sugar to be consumed, so by the end product, you will hardly be ingesting any of it. Apple cider vinegar has between three and five calories for each tablespoon, and you only need a little to achieve the benefits you desire.

In other words, you end up with a great drink that has little to no sugar or calories. Actually, one major advantage to consuming apple cider vinegar is the positive impact on your blood sugar levels, as mentioned earlier. It helps them stay stable, reducing hypoglycemia and diabetes risks.

Apple Cider Vinegar as a Disinfectant:

Vinegar is proven to have abilities to fight fungus and to kill bad pathogens and bacteria. Throughout history, people have used it to clean their bodies, homes, and to prevent fungus. In modern day, people are still using apple cider vinegar extensively to clean their houses and bodies.

History and Overview of Apple Cider Vinegar

Did you know that apple cider vinegar has been ingested for over 2,000 years? Records of history prove that people have been fermenting apple juice into vinegar since around 5,000 BC or earlier.

Cleansing the Body:

Throughout time, apple cider vinegar has been put to use as a circulation stimulant a detoxification aid for the liver, a way to improve immunity, cleanse the lymph nodes, and to purify the blood. Actually, Hippocrates was known to prescribe apple cider vinegar for colds and coughs, mixed with a little honey.

How Else Did the Ancients Use Apple Cider Vinegar?

Vinegar, especially apple cider vinegar, is one of our greatest gifts from nature and the history of the liquid proves this. This vinegar is truly natural. All alcoholic beverages, whether made from plain sugar, rice, dates, grapes, or apples, will turn into vinegar after exposed to the air.

The bacteria present in the air is always there, and it converts alcohol from beer, wine, and cider into the previously mentioned acetic acid. This is what causes vinegar to taste so sour and sharp. Given this information, it's safe to assume that humans have been using vinegar since before they started recording that use.

The Recorded History of Vinegar:

The recorded history of vinegar begins at 5,000 BC. The Babylonians started using date palm fruit for creating vinegar and wine. This was used to pickle items, preserve food, and just to eat it. Residues from vinegar have been discovered in urns from ancient Egypt as old as 3,000 BC. In addition, the history of recorded vinegar use is present in texts from 1,200 BC in China.

Biblical Use of Vinegar:

In the times of the Bible, vinegar was being drunk for energy, used for medicine, and put on foods as flavoring. The liquid is mentioned in the new and old testaments of the bible. For instance, Ruth, after working hard in the barley fields, was given bread and vinegar by Boaz.

Vinegar and the Military:

The history of vinegar shows plenty of examples of the usefulness of the substance to soldiers. Vinegar, diluted in water, has been given as an energizing and strengthening tonic throughout history by the military.

"Posca" and Roman Soldiers:

Soldiers in ancient Roman times referred to this drink as "posca" and drank it often, just as the Japanese samurai did. Adding this substance to ordinary water also kills off infectious agents within the liquid, making it safer to drink.

Speeding up Healing:

Across history, vinegar has been recognized for its antiseptic nature and was used to disinfect and clean wounds of soldiers, speeding up their healing. Apple cider vinegar was also used in this way throughout the civil war in America, along with the times of World War One.

The Dissolving Abilities of Vinegar:

Vinegar has a well-known dissolving power that was used by Hannibal, the Carthaginian general when he went with elephants across the Alps and invaded Italy around the year 218 BC. This liquid was poured over hot stones to break them up, allowing his men to proceed and march across.

Vinegar and Louis XIII:

Louis XIII of France (who lived between 1601 and 1643) is said to have paid over a million Francs for vinegar so he could cool his army's cannons in a battle. Vinegar was applied to the cannons (made of hot iron) and cooled them down, preventing rust and cleaning the metal surface.

Vinegar in the Middle Ages:

Another use of apple cider vinegar in history was the Middle Ages. In addition to abrasive substances like sand, vinegar can be (and was) used to polish and clean armor.

Surprising Uses of Vinegar in History:

Cleopatra and Vinegar:

Around the year 40 BC, history says that the queen of Egypt, Cleopatra, won a bet with Mark Anthony, the Roman General, when she dissolved an expensive pearl in a glass of vinegar and drank it down. She had wagered that she could offer a feast for them both that cost a fortune.

Vinegar and Alchemy:

European alchemists were no stranger to vinegar around the Middle Ages. They poured vinegar over the lead, making a sweet substance known as sugar of lead. This substance was put to use for sweetening and smoothing out the taste of harsh cider.

Sadly, lead acetate is a poisonous subject and lead to the death of many cider drinkers in Europe around this time. Please note that you should never store vinegar in containers of crystal glass, iron, copper, or lead.

The Bubonic Plague:

From the 1300s to the 1700s, many cities in Europe were affected by the awful bubonic plague. At this time, around 50 million people perished due to this disease, which spread to men from rats and fleas.

By the year 1721, the plague had hit cities in France so hard that it was impossible to decently bury all of the dead. In order to solve this situation, authorities in the country let condemned convicts out of prison so they could help bury the bodies.

According to historical accords, most people died, but a particular group of convicted thieves survived by drinking garlic-infused vinegar every day in large amounts. Due to this, garlic-steeped vinegar is still known as Four Thieves Vinegar today.

European aristocrats held sponges soaked in vinegar to their noises to ward off the harmful odors of raw sewage and outdoor garbage in the 17th and 18th centuries. Vinaigrettes (small boxes) were carried around with these sponges inside, and many people stored these in their walking canes in special compartments.

Vinegar and Commercial Use:

In the late 1300s, some vintners in France came up with a method for creating vinegar known as the Orleans method. This involved using oak barrels to ferment the vinegar, then siphoning the liquid off using a spigot located on the barrel bottom.

About 15 percent of this liquid remained behind and had floating on top the famous "Mother of vinegar" along with concentrated bacteria. Then, a new batch of wine or cider was added to this barrel, which the remaining vinegar jump started for fermentation.

This group of vintners in France started a master vinegar creator's guild, using their Orleans method, and were able to supply the market of lucrative vinegar making.

Vinegar as Flavoring:

The industry of vinegar in the area was flourishing at the time of the Renaissance. Many kinds of vinegar flavored with flowers, fruits, herbs, and spices came out around this time, and around the 18th century, more than a hundred types existed.

Common Myths about Apple Cider Vinegar

Myth #1: Apple cider vinegar has identical nutrients as a normal apple.

Even though apple cider vinegar does come from apples being fermented, hard cider does too, and this doesn't lead people to drink it to gain more health. Apples have Vitamin C and fiber, but these are not present in apple cider vinegar. As mentioned, potassium does exist in the liquid, but only about 5 percent of how much there is of a real apple.

Myth #2: Apple cider vinegar offers no health advantages.

A lot of people believe that apple cider vinegar cannot possibly have so many health benefits. As you will see throughout this book, it clearly does!

Myth #3: All Apple cider vinegar is created equal.

When it comes to cheap brands to more expensive, better organic types, it appears as though nearly all food companies are trying to get the apple cider vinegar kick and profit from it.

However, there are differences between types of apple cider vinegar. The clear types have been thoroughly processed and filtered, sacrificing some of its amazing health benefits. Instead, go for the murky-looking, brown variety if possible.

Myth #4: You can only use it to drink or eat.

With the health advantages touted for apple cider vinegar, it appears as though this is as far as its benefits go. However, it's a very versatile liquid. Apple cider vinegar is great for cleaning the house because of its antimicrobial functions. Use it to wipe your counters at home, and you'll be amazed.

Myth #5: You should never use apple cider vinegar topically.

Due to its strong smell and acidic components, apple cider vinegar seems as though it would be too harsh to use on your skin, but this is not the case. It shouldn't be used to replace your facial moisturizer, but when you mix it with water, you can use it for a facial toner to clear makeup and dirt away from your face.

To do this, simply apply the apple cider vinegar to your face using a cotton swab and keep it there for 10 minutes, then rinse it off. This mixture can be used to replace your ordinary face wash, but only do it about three times each week.

Myth #6: Apple cider vinegar is the only type of vinegar that is healthy.

Apple cider vinegar is very healthy and is considered the best of the best, but some health advantages can be reaped from other types of vinegar, as well. Since all vinegar has acetic acid in it, plain white vinegar and balsamic vinegar can also be beneficial.

Myth #7: Apple cider vinegar is only fit for human use.

Your pet can actually benefit from this liquid, as well. In fact, some holistic veterinarians use it to fix itchy ears and skin in animals. Just use equal parts water and apple cider vinegar, then spray it onto your dog or cat's itchy spots to bring relief. Never spray this onto open wounds.

Myth #8: It doesn't taste good.

Some people like the taste of apple cider vinegar and others don't. It's true that taste is an individual preference and is very subjective, but you don't have to take apple cider vinegar by itself. You can mix it with melted coconut or olive oil and herbs to create a tasty salad dressing or mix it into a fruit smoothie.

Later on in the book, we will cover some specific recipes you can use to get the benefits of apple cider vinegar without drinking it by itself.

Chapter 2: How to Make Raw Apple Cider Vinegar

When apple season comes around, it's time to create your own apple cider vinegar at home. If you can't find a locally grown source for apples where you live, you can just buy a bag from your local store (make sure they're organic though).

Why Make Your Own?

Raw, unpasteurized apple cider vinegar costs a lot, so you can save money by making your own at home. Your average quart of the liquid will cost you around $5 at the majority of health grocery stores.

You can create an entire gallon or more for this price, or even cheaper using apple scraps that would've been thrown away anyway.

Which Apples to Use:

You might be wondering which types of apples to use to make your homemade apple cider vinegar. The truth is that a mix of apples is what will create the healthiest and best-tasting type. If you have never done this before, try out the ratios below to create your very first batch, and you can mix it as you prefer later on.

- 50 Percent sweet types of apples, such as Red Delicious, Fuji, or Golden Delicious.

- About 35 percent sharp apples, like Liberty, Northern Spy, or Liberty.

- 15 percent bitter apples, like Cortland, Porter's Perfection, or Newtown.

In some places, bitter apples might be hard to find at the store. If you encounter this problem, you can use 60 percent sweet apples and use 40 percent sharp apples. The flavor won't end up being as complex, but it will work just fine. If you just have one type of apple tree at home, though, you can just use that type to create your apple cider vinegar.

Making Raw ACV at Home:

This recipe will make about a gallon of apple cider vinegar but can be adjusted to suit your needs. For example, use half to get half the amount, and twice the amount to get twice as much.

Plus, you can make as much as you want without having to go buy more. Who can argue with that type of convenience? When you make your own, you get to control the quality, the process of making it, and how much to create. Keep reading to find out how to make this amazing liquid to help your health.

Your Ingredients List:

- Five big apples, or the leftovers from 10 apples.

- Clean, filtered water.

- Organic sugar or raw honey (1 cup).

- 1 Gallon jar made of glass.

- One large rubber band.

- A cheesecloth for straining.

Instructions for making Raw ACV:

Before you start this process, you need to create hard apple cider, first. The alcohol from this mixture is what causes acetic acid to form, which is what contributes to the sour taste and health benefits of apple cider vinegar. Then, you're ready to follow these steps:

1. Make sure your apples are washed, then chop it up into coarse pieces of about an inch across. The seeds, stems, and cores can be included in this.

2. Put your coarsely chopped apple pieces in your jar (after making sure it's clean). Make sure you aren't brewing this cider in steel pots since the acidic mixture can cause heavy metals to leach and harm your body. The apples should fill the jar at least halfway or more. Add more scraps and chunks until the jar is at least halfway full.

3. Pour water over the scraps and apple chunks until they are covered, and your container is almost full, but leave some room toward the top. Make sure the water is room temperature.

4. Stir the sugar and honey into the container until it dissolves completely. Cover your jar with a cheesecloth and hold it in place with a big rubber band.

5. Leave this jar sitting on your counter for a week or two, but remember to mix it gently a couple of times each day. You will notice bubbles forming. This is the sugar being fermented into an alcohol substance. You will also notice this in the smell of the mixture.

6. You will know that the hard cider is ready when the chunks of apple don't float anymore and have sunk to the jar's bottom. If the apple chunks still have not sunk down after 14 days but your mix smells like alcohol, move onto the following step.

7. Strain the apple chunks out, pouring the resulting liquid to a clean jar or multiple smaller jars. Then, cover this with a new cheesecloth, tying it on using a rubber band.

8. Leave this mixture on your counter for another three to four weeks so that the alcohol can get transformed into acetic acid by the acetic acid bacteria. Seeing some sediment at the jar's bottom is to be expected. You will see the mother culture start to form on the top of the liquid.

9. You can taste your mixture after three weeks to see if it's done If the taste seems right for you, strain the mix and keep it in clean jugs or mason jars. If the taste doesn't seem right after four weeks, leave it for seven days and make another attempt.

10. If you forget about it and it's left too long, you may strain the mix and dilute it with water until it reaches the level you want.

This mixture can be used as you pleased but be sure to store it way from sunlight or extreme temperatures.

Raw, organic apple cider vinegar will not go bad, but another mother will form atop it if it's left for too long, so keep that in mind. If this does happen, it's fine, you will just need to restrain it and dilute again if it's too strong tasting.

Remember that your homemade vinegar isn't just useful for the kitchen. You can also use it in the bath (add two cups to a tub full of water) to help your body detox. You may also use it as a compress when you get a bruise or sprain, as people once did before ice was more common.

Remember to use Non-Pasteurized:

As mentioned before, apple cider vinegar that has been pasteurized doesn't give you the same health advantages as the raw stuff in terms of enzymes, probiotics, or vitamins. If you decide to go through the process of making your own apple cider vinegar, make sure it's raw.

Don't use Plastic Packaged Apple Cider Vinegar:

Another issue with apple cider vinegar that has been pasteurized is that it's often packaged in a plastic bottle. The acidic apple cider vinegar will leach chemicals from the plastic into the fluid. If you make your own or buy it at the store, always make sure it's a glass bottle.

<u>More Uses for Apple Cider Vinegar to Know about:</u>

The uses for this liquid are seemingly endless. You can make a master tonic with it, which is a natural anti-viral and anti-flu agent. Apple cider vinegar is also an important component of bone broth. Let's look at some other uses for this liquid.

Polishing Wood:

Apple cider vinegar can actually be used to condition wood. Just mix half a cup of the fluid with half a cup of oil (such as olive or vegetable), and it will create a great furniture polish for removing water stains and treating surfaces.

Treating Digestion Issues:

If you drink a bit before eating, apple cider vinegar will treat digestion issues such as indigestion and bloating.

Curing Warts:

Although the scientific proof for this is not very vast, there are countless testimonials online that swear by using apple cider vinegar to cure warts. Before going to bed, soak a cotton swab with some diluted apple cider vinegar and paste it in place overnight. Your wart may throb and swell, then fall off after a couple weeks.

An Alternative to Harsh Chemicals:

A lot of people don't like the idea of spraying their home with harsh chemicals. Get rid of the commercial stuff and make your own with two parts water to one-part vinegar. You may add some essential oils for scent and extra disinfectant properties.

A Word from the Experts:

Dr. Sandi Rogers, a naturopath CEO of a College of Traditional Medicine in Australia, has been studying the healing benefits of apple cider vinegar for over three decades and believes that it's an impressive medicine. Rogers believes that the superfood status of apple cider vinegar is due to its high content of minerals.

Since minerals are so foundational to wellbeing and health (not vitamins, as some believe), taking this liquid each day can help you immensely, especially with mineral absorption from your diet.

How much to Use:

Use regular, small amounts, such as a couple teaspoons dissolved in some water. Swish it around in your mouth in order to activate your salivary glands.

The Safety of Apple Cider Vinegar:

Many may wonder, is apple cider vinegar completely safe? Admittedly, the risks and benefits of this liquid aren't completely known yet, so if you have any doubts, your illnesses should always be managed and treated with a professional of medical status.

Again, the uglier the vinegar, the healthier it is. For most people, drinking apple cider vinegar straight will be too sour to handle and may even burn the esophagus. For this reason, dilute it with water. If you still can't stand the sourness, add some raw honey to the water before drinking.

All About "The Mother"

You have heard us mention "the mother" a couple of times, but what exactly does this mean? Again, it's crucial to realize that apple cider vinegar can vary greatly in quality. In order to get the best of the best apple cider vinegar, make sure the mother is still intact in the bottle.

The mother ensures that the vinegar still has its advantageous components, such as probiotics. The mother probiotics are the cloudy strands within the vinegar where all of the health benefits come from.

AMAZING Health Benefits of Apple Cider Vinegar

After reading this far, you should have a pretty good understanding of why you should use apple cider vinegar on a daily basis. But here are some more health benefits to be aware of:

- **Body Detox:** Raw, unfiltered apple cider vinegar is a lymphatic and liver tonic which helps your body clean itself out, balancing the pH, stimulating bowel motility, cardiovascular stimulation, and lymphatic drainage. In other words, it really helps your body get clean!

  Usually, when we hear the word acid, associated with vinegar, we automatically assume that acid is bad. However, for this, acid is very good. Similar to the way lemon juice contains citric acid which helps lemon water detoxify your body, the acetic acid in apple cider vinegar also has an incredible alkalizing effect on you. This aids in weight loss efforts, energy levels, and many other things.

- **Teeth Whitening:** Apple cider vinegar has a high pH level which is useful for removing stains, not just from your kitchen counters, but from your teeth. Just take your first finger, dip it in some apple cider vinegar and rub it onto your teeth, allowing it to sit for one to two minutes.

- **Treating Heartburn and Acid Reflux:** One of the main reasons that people get acid reflux and uncomfortable heartburn is a stomach pH that isn't balanced enough, lacking probiotics and important enzymes. Luckily, apple cider vinegar has plenty of these essential nutrients.

How should this be taken? Just add a tablespoon of the liquid to a full glass of water and make sure to drink it down five to 10 minutes before eating. This will relieve your heartburn and acid reflux symptoms.

Killing Candida: Countless people across the globe struggle with yeast and candida. This can lead to digestive problems, UTIs, a lack of energy, and bad breath. Thankfully, apple cider vinegar has properties to help this.

The probiotics present in apple cider vinegar will help promote probiotic growth to kill this harmful yeast. Another way to help this is to stop eating sugar altogether.

- **Keep your pH Levels Balanced:** Apple cider vinegar, as stated a few times already, is full of acetic acid, which has an alkalizing effect on your body.

Keeping your pH in balance will help reduce the risk of cancer and improve your energy levels.

- **Supports Metabolism:** A research study done by the *Journal of Diabetes Care* discovered that you could promote weight loss by ingesting apple cider vinegar. A few different reasons exist for this, but one main reason is that apple cider vinegar reduces cravings for sugar and helps detox your body.

  Another useful study discovered that adding acetic acid to the diet reduced the body fat of rats by up to 10 percent. Another study done in 2005 discovered that consuming vinegar along with a meal with high carbs reduced the drinking and eating of participants by 200 to 275 calories within a day.

- **Ease your Sunburn:** Sunburn can be very uncomfortable, but apple cider vinegar is here to the rescue again! Just add a cup of the liquid to a mildly temperature bath with some lavender essential oil and a quarter cup of coconut oil. This will help your sunburn not only feel better in the moment, but heal overall.

- **Balance your Blood Sugar:** Studies have shown that acetic acid helps to balance blood sugar, improving insulin responses and sensitivity.

- **Soothing Inflammation and Swelling:** Raw, organic apple cider vinegar has potassium in it, which helps to reduce inflammation and swelling. This can be used to treat poison ivy.

- **Get Fleas off your Dog or Cat:** An apple cider vinegar solution can help remove fleas from your pets. Just mix together 50 percent water with 50 percent apple cider vinegar and wash your pet with the mix. Do this once per day for a few weeks, and your pet will be free from fleas.

- **Help Allergies:** Yet another great way to use apple cider vinegar is to treat allergies. Apple cider vinegar can help to break the mucous up in your body. In addition, it clears sinuses and supports a healthy immune system. You can drink it a few times a day to cure your allergy symptoms.

- **Kill Toenail Fungus:** The antifungal and antibacterial components of apple cider vinegar will help kill toenail and skin fungus. Just rub some apple cider vinegar onto the affected area a couple times a day.

- **Fight Eczema:** As mentioned, apple cider vinegar has a high pH level, making it great for curing skin problems. Next time your eczema pops up, rub the liquid onto the affected area or wash with it. You can also use essential oils and coconut oil to heal further.

- **Fight Varicose Veins:** This miracle liquid is great for fighting varicose veins. This is possible because apple cider vinegar improves your circulation, is anti-inflammatory, and supports the health of your vein walls, reducing the bulging veins. Just mix the liquid with some witch hazel, then rub it onto your veins to see improvement.

- **A Sore Throat Cure:** Due to its probiotic properties and vitamins, apple cider vinegar is a great way to cure your sore throat or cold. Take a spoonful diluted in water thrice daily to have this effect.

- **Fight Odors:** Harmful yeast and bad bacteria are a couple of the main causes of bad body odors. Your armpits often stay damp throughout the day, leading to bad bacteria and the smell we associate with that area.

Just dabbing some of your homemade, raw apple cider vinegar under this area can help to neutralize odors by killing off the yeast there.

Scientific Backed Claims of Apple Cider Vinegar

Even after reading this far into the book, you might still be skeptical about whether apple cider vinegar really can offer all these amazing benefits. So for this section, we are going to focus primarily on scientifically-backed claims of the health benefits of apple cider vinegar.

Fosters Healthy Cholesterol in the Body:

Apple cider vinegar can not only support your body's cholesterol levels, but research has proven that it also protects your body from oxidation or arterial damage, which high cholesterol can lead to. WebMD mentions a study done in the mid 2000's that provided evidence for apple cider vinegar lowering cholesterol numbers

Reduces Water Retention:

We've already mentioned that apple cider vinegar is a helpful weight loss aid, but did you know that it also reduces water retention? Paired with its abilities to increase your metabolism and suppress your appetite, this is a pretty amazing combination for those looking to shed some extra weight. The Journal of Agricultural and Food Chemistry found out in 2010 that apple cider vinegar reduced water retention in mice.

Blocks Starch Digestion in the Body:

Research has proven that apple cider vinegar contains powerful anti-glycemic compounds that help your body support healthy levels of blood sugar. In addition, apple cider vinegar blocks starch digestion in your body (partially), which is known to raise blood sugar levels. A 2004 study done by "Diabetes Care" found a link between improved sensitivity to insulin and the consumption of vinegar, especially during high-carb meals.

Antioxidants:

Apple cider vinegar has multiple antioxidants which will help you stay physically healthy and keep your body running in top shape. Biochem Pharmacol published a paper in 1994 that discovered high antioxidant activity in the acetic acid present in apple cider vinegar.

Helps you Absorb Vegetable Nutrients:

We've already mentioned that the acetic acid present in this vinegar helps your body absorb crucial nutrients from your food, but did you know that adding some of this to your salad can specifically help you get the most out of your vegetables and leafy greens?

Researchers in Japan, working for Biosci Biotechnol chemistry found that dietary vinegar helped the intestinal absorption of calcium in rats in 1999

Fights Diabetes:

The next incredible advantage that apple cider vinegar offers is that it can become part of a great plan to help diabetes. Multiple studies have discovered that apple cider vinegar can lower your levels of glucose, meaning that it's an effective treatment for those suffering from type 2 diabetes.

A study done in 2007 by the University of Arizona discovered that drinking two tablespoons of the liquid in addition to 30 grams of cheese right before going to sleep could decrease fasting levels of blood sugar by 4 to 6 percent!

Another study done by *Diabetes Care,* the medical journal, discovered that taking just two tablespoons of the liquid before a meal can decrease levels of blood sugar by 6 percent! That's because the liquid has been proven to reduce A1C levels and balance out levels of blood sugar, which helps diabetics immensely.

In addition, if you eat and typically experience a spike in blood sugar afterward, the vinegar can help your energy levels rise again.

Chapter 3: Detoxing with Apple Cider Vinegar

We have already covered some of the incredible benefits of apple cider vinegar, including its ability to lower your blood pressure, treat acid reflux, and support the overall health of your gut. In addition, the acetic acid within apple cider vinegar helps to support healthy digestive function, and only a little is needed to reap these benefits.

Let's look next at one of the greatest benefits of apple cider vinegar, its role in effective weight loss.

<u>Natural Weight Loss using Apple Cider Vinegar:</u>

Being overweight is embarrassing in addition to being uncomfortable. If you have been trying and trying to lose weight and keep it off, you're probably ready to try something completely new.

Apple Cider Vinegar and Dieting:

ACV (apple cider vinegar) is a well-known natural remedy and is used by countless people to both cure and prevent common ailments. In addition, this liquid holds a crucial spot in the world of dieting. Scientific research along with personal experiences have proven that apple cider vinegar can, in fact, help you reach your ideal weight.

The Long-Term Answer:

Just treating the symptoms of a problem, without going deeper, will not provide a lasting solution. Apple cider vinegar is a substance that can target your weight problem from a holistic perspective, offering a long-term answer instead of a quick fix.

Proof and Research about ACV and Weight Loss:

This chapter is here to help you know how apple cider vinegar works, along with how you can use it day to day to improve your overall health and lose that extra weight.

One of the most interesting studies done on how this liquid can aid weight loss was done in the year 2009 by *Bioscience, Biotechnology, and Biochemistry*. This study found that drinking a couple of tablespoons of apple cider vinegar for a few months caused participants to lose significant amounts of body fat and waist circumference.

How Does Apple Cider Vinegar Help Your Body Shed Weight?

Apple cider vinegar comes from apples that are crushed, distilled, and finally fermented, as we went over earlier in the book. This results in acetic acid, a liquid that taps into some important physiological functions and supports the healthy loss of extra weight on your body. Let's look at some of the other reasons it helps you lose weight.

The Appetite Suppressant Effect:

Apple cider vinegar, first and foremost, helps you to eat less, causing your body to feel satisfied sooner than it normally would while eating. One study that showed this beyond doubt was done in 2005. The participants who ate their bread with some vinegar got full faster than the others who ate just bread.

The higher amount of acetic acid they consumed, the fuller the participants felt over the course of the study.

Blood Sugar Control for Weight Loss:

Apple cider vinegar helps to control your levels of blood sugar, as mentioned previously. It prevents those uncontrollable spikes in sugar and the crashes that lead you to want to snack in between the main meals of the day.

Once your blood sugar levels are stable, you will find it easier to eat just when you're hungry and stay with your diet. The study mentioned before also kept track of blood sugar levels with both the control group and vinegar group.

Study participants who consumed apple cider vinegar had much lower blood glucose levels after their meal. In other words, there wasn't the spike that usually comes after a high-carb meal. In addition, the ones who consumed larger doses of apple cider vinegar were still benefiting from the impact an hour and a half after they ate.

It helps to Prevent the Accumulation of Fat:

Apple cider vinegar helps to stimulate your body's metabolism function which helps you burn more fat faster. In addition, it has a lot of enzyme and organic acids that help you burn more fat by speeding your metabolism up.

Insulin Secretion and Apple Cider Vinegar:

Did you know that insulin plays a role in your body's storage of fat? It's true. Insulin is closely related to your levels of blood sugar, and the secretion of this hormone is disrupted in those who suffer from diabetes (type 2).

Some scientists suggested that apple cider vinegar could work very similarly to diabetic drugs, controlling this disease. For helping to cure your diabetes, diet is highly important. Do plenty of research into the foods and spices you should be consuming.

Apple Cider Vinegar's Detoxing Effect and Weight Loss:

When your body sheds harmful toxins, metabolism and digestion become much more efficient than before. Apple cider vinegar flushes out your body, allowing it to make the best use of the nutrients you eat. It also has high levels of insoluble fiber, improving bowel movements and absorbing toxins.

<u>Which Type of Apple Cider Vinegar to Use for Losing Weight:</u>

We've gone over this for other health benefits of apple cider vinegar, but it's especially crucial for weight loss. When you are using the liquid for this specific purpose, it must be raw and unprocessed. Better yet, use the kind you are making at home.

You should know by now that you should only be using apple cider vinegar that still has the mother intact to get the best benefits possible.

Avoiding Pesticides:

Apples are one of the most heavily sprayed fruits out there, when it comes to pesticides, making organic choices very important! You must purchase unfiltered, unprocessed, raw apple cider vinegar to get the benefits you seek and to lose weight, or just make your own.

Brand isn't as Important as Other Factors:

You may be wondering which brand of apple cider vinegar to use for weight loss, but brand doesn't matter as much as some other considerations. Any apple cider vinegar brand that is organic, unfiltered, and unpasteurized may be used for this reason.

One very common brand of organic apple cider vinegar is Bragg. You can buy this on the Internet, in health food stores, or in ordinary supermarkets, sometimes.

Don't worry about the apple cider vinegar not being pasteurized, since vinegar has a high enough level of acidity to kill off E. Coli and other harmful bacteria. Keep in mind that many doctors say that pregnant women shouldn't consume unpasteurized foods.

Steps for Using ACV to Lose Weight:

For those who don't like or are not accustomed to the flavor and impact of apple cider vinegar, you can start by including the liquid gradually in your diet, being careful not to use too much. This will prevent adverse effects.

How to Start:

You can begin by adding just a teaspoon of the vinegar to a glass of water, drinking this mixture at least one time per day. You can slowly increase the amount every time and how often you drink it.

The Optimal Amount to Drink:

According to studies on apple cider vinegar and weight loss, the ideal amount to consume per day is two tablespoons, diluted in water. Dilution is important because the liquid is highly acidic and dilution helps to protect your stomach lining, throat, and teeth.

Using a Straw:

Don't ever drink apple cider vinegar undiluted, this will cause you more harm than anything else. You may drink the diluted mix of apple cider vinegar and water using a straw. This will keep your tooth enamel safe.

Using Honey with Apple Cider Vinegar:

Some people will discover that the apple cider vinegar taste is hard to stand. In order to make the flavor more tolerable, you may add a little honey to it. The honey will mix better if you use warm water.

Mixing apple cider vinegar and honey have benefits for your health, and it also tastes great. If you are aiming to lose weight, try not to use too much honey as sugar can get in the way of weight loss.

Adding Apple Cider Vinegar to Food:

- **Soups**: Apple cider vinegar can be used with certain foods and goes especially well with meat or bean soups. Just keep in mind that you should add the vinegar to your food after it has cooled. This will prevent the loss of nutrients to the heat.

- **Salads**: Apple cider vinegar is a popular dressing for salads and tastes especially great with olive oil and herbs added.

- **Pickling**: For those who enjoy pickles or similar flavors, you can use apple cider vinegar to pickle cucumbers or other vegetables.

- **Herbal Tea**: For those who don't mind the taste of apple cider vinegar, you can add it to your herbal teas to get the health benefits. This book will go over some other recipes later on.

How Often Should You Drink it?

In order to jump-start your metabolism and get the benefits of feeling full, some say that you must drink diluted apple cider vinegar an hour before eating to help you lose weight and improve digestion.

Morning Vinegar:

Some swear by drinking their apple cider vinegar right when they wake up and have empty stomachs. But others prefer not to do this. If you aren't comfortable drinking it without food in your stomach, you can do it after meals.

After Meals:

If you're more comfortable consuming apple cider vinegar after meals, you can do this two to three times per day. If you feel nausea or burning in your stomach, reduce how much you're taking.

Taking Breaks:

Some people recommend not consuming apple cider vinegar every single day and making sure to take breaks every month or so. As you can see, it all depends on what suits you best.

Possible Side Effects of Apple Cider Vinegar:

ACV is considered generally safe for human consumption, but as with all traditional remedies, you should take some precautions to make sure you're safe. Too much apple cider vinegar could lead to lowered levels of potassium in the body, causing osteoporosis.

But this effect happened to someone who drank 8 oz. of ACV every day for multiple years in a row. As you can see, we recommend jutting a couple tablespoons diluted every day, which is more than safe to consume regularly.

As said before, acidic items like apple cider vinegar can lead to weaker tooth enamel, so to prevent that, just rinse the mouth out with water each time you drink the apple cider vinegar mixture. Use a straw, too, to prevent tooth problems. You might also wish to refrain from brushing your teeth right after taking your apple cider vinegar mix.

Asking your Doctor about Interactions:

Apple cider vinegar may interact with diabetes medications, heart medications, laxatives, or diuretics. If you're on any meds, make sure you ask your physician before you decide to drink apple cider vinegar regularly.

Why is Apple Cider Vinegar Superior to Other Types for Losing Weight?

Apple cider vinegar is believed to be the best choice when it comes to weight loss, due to all of the health advantages it offers. It will clean your body, offering anti-microbial effects.

Considering the fact that it can aid high blood pressure, heart issues, diabetes, digestion, acid reflux, and possibly even kidney stones, it's obvious why apple cider vinegar is the best type of vinegar to use for health reasons.

<u>What Should You Expect Using Apple Cider Vinegar To Lose Weight?</u>

Apple cider vinegar should not be expected to give you an instant cure for a weight problem. The changes you see will happen on a gradual basis, but they will be permanent.

Patience is Key:

Remember to be patient, letting it work. At times, losing a pound per month and keeping it off is the real path to success. Don't get impatient and give up!

Other Factors in Weight Loss:

Also, keep in mind that the rate at which you lose your weight does depend on your other lifestyle habits, like genetics, stress, nutrition, and how much you exercise.

<u>Making the Apple Cider Vinegar Work Better and Faster:</u>

To get the fastest and best results, you have to combine this remedy with other proven methods. That way, the apple cider vinegar will work along with these other changes and give you the results you're hoping for.

Avoid Processed Foods:

If you're hoping to lose weight, you must avoid processed foods, unhealthy fats, and sugar. All of these will counteract the effects of the vinegar.

Find some Exercise You Enjoy:

Even moving moderately up to five times each week can help you speed up your metabolism and lose weight faster. Start by walking for 10 minutes each day and work your way up.

Potassium-Rich Foods:

If you eat foods that have plenty of potassium, this mineral can lower your blood pressure and reduce your stress levels. Each more spinach, avocados, sweet potatoes, and bananas to get this effect.

Beauty Benefits of Apple Cider Vinegar:

Apple cider vinegar isn't just good for your health and cleaning, it also has beauty benefits that help you look better! Let's look at some of those now.

Beauty Benefit #1: Use it to Brighten Your Nails.

Stained or yellow nails can be a bit embarrassing, and this occurs from smoking or other tasks. It can happen after working with dyes or chemicals or just bad habits. Whatever your reason for having stained nails, apple cider vinegar can help whiten them.

The acetic and malic acids present in apple cider vinegar will reduce the stains on your nails and also help to treat nail infections, which can lead to discoloration. Here are the steps for cleaning your nails with apple cider vinegar:

- Put half a cup of lukewarm water and half a cup of apple cider vinegar into a bowl wide enough to soak your hands in.

- Soak your yellowed nails in the mixture for up to a half hour, then rise.

- Use coconut or olive oil to massage into each nail.

- You can do this twice a day until your nails brighten up.

Beauty Benefit #2: Keep Pimples and Acne Away.

If you have a pimple problem, apple cider vinegar can help with that, as well. The liquid has antibacterial and antiseptic properties that help keep pimples away by freeing your pores of dust particles, oil, and bacteria.

It also helps your skin regain a healthy pH balance, which helps to keep breakouts away. Here are the steps for using apple cider vinegar to treat and prevent acne:

- Mix two parts water with one-part organic apple cider vinegar in a bowl.

- Wet some cotton balls with the liquid, putting it on your affected area.

- Let this sit for 15 minutes and then rinse it.

- You can do this up to three times per day for four days.

Beauty Benefit #3: Use it for Skin Toning.

People with oily skin can benefit from apple cider vinegar due to its properties that work as an astringent. Apple cider vinegar contains properties that help get more blood flow going on your face, minimizing pores.

After a short time, your skin will start looking much better. Just stick with it faithfully so you can start to see the results you hope for. This, in combination with its antiseptic properties, it will help your skin look awesome. Just follow these steps to get the benefits:

- Mix half a cup of distilled water with half a cup of apple cider vinegar. You can add some essential oil too, like ylang-ylang or lavender, just use a few drops.

- Put this mixture on your face with a cotton ball, allowing it to sit three minutes.

- Rinse your face off using cold water. This can be done two times each day but make sure you shake the liquid before applying it.

For those with average skin, you can use two parts water with one-part apple cider vinegar for your toner, but if your skin is very sensitive, more water is suggested. Always make sure you test this out on a small area of your skin before using.

Keep in mind that when you use this liquid, the vinegar smell may stay on your skin for a bit, but does fade once the toner dries.

Beauty Benefit #4: Get Rid of Razor Burn and Bumps.

The irritated, small bumps you get on your skin after shaving are not only unattractive, but they can be painful. In order to help solve this issue, you may utilize apple cider vinegar.

The anti-inflammatory compounds in the apple cider vinegar will help soothe your irritated areas, reducing itching and inflammation. In addition to this, the acetic acid present in apple cider vinegar will soften your skin while keeping infections away, helping your ingrown hairs disappear.

In order to utilize this wonderful natural remedy for razor bumps and burn, follow these steps:

- Smear a small amount of honey over your razor burn, letting it sit for five minutes or so.

- Rinse the honey off using cool water.

- Using a cotton swab, put apple cider vinegar on the affected area, allowing it to try out on its own.

- This treatment can be repeated three times daily until your razor burn goes away.

Keep in mind that if you have sensitive skin, diluting the apple cider vinegar will be safer for you.

Beauty Benefit #5: Get rid of Teeth Stains.

If your teeth are yellow and stained, it can be embarrassing, making you self-conscious, but you can use apple cider vinegar to help clean them up. Discoloration comes from drinking too much coffee or smoking.

Apple cider vinegar's acetic acid content will help get rid of this yellow, stained surface, destroying harmful mouth bacteria and contributing to a healthier mouth all around. Here's how to use it for this:

- Mix a tablespoon of water with a tablespoon of apple cider vinegar and use it as a mouthwash in the morning and at night.

Beauty Benefit #6: Get rid of Dandruff.

Although dandruff isn't dangerous, it doesn't look very nice and can lead to embarrassment. This problem is worst during the winter because the air tends to be so dry.

Dandruff leads to dead, oily skin pieces on your hair and scalp. This may eventually cause a scaly, itchy head and even shoulders covered in dandruff flakes. ACV has antifungal compounds that restore your scalp's pH balance, cleaning out your hair follicles and clogged pores.

Here's how to use apple cider vinegar as a remedy for dandruff:

- Mix two tablespoons of water with two tablespoons of apple cider vinegar.

- Mix 15 drops of the liquid of tea tree oil.

- Spread this liquid onto your head, massaging for about five minutes, then let it sit for five minutes.

- Your hair can be rinsed and washed with shampoo as normal, and this treatment may be used three times each week until your issue is resolved.

Beauty Benefit #7: Make your Feet Smell Better.

Smelly feet, or foot odor, is an issue that is quite common but can still be unpleasant and embarrassing both for you and your friends. The antimicrobial properties of apple cider vinegar can help to disinfect and clean your feet, killing off bacteria that causes this odor.

Here are the steps you must take to kill foot odor using apple cider vinegar:

- Add five cups of warm water with a cup of apple cider vinegar.

- Let your feet sit in this liquid for up to 15 minutes.

- After you let them sit, wash them with water and soap.

- This can be used at home every day for about a month.

Beauty Benefit #8: Help your Sunburn Heal.

The sun is good for us in moderation, but when you're outside underneath it for too long, it can cause a painful sunburn. This turns your skin painful and red from the damage. In extreme cases, you might even get blisters.

Apple cider vinegar has been used for many years to cure this issue. Due to its natural astringent abilities, apple cider vinegar helps to speed healing and soothe the burning feeling. It also reduces inflammation and irritation.

Here's how to use apple cider vinegar to soothe your sunburn:

- Mix some cool water with an equal amount of apple cider vinegar, massaging this mixture onto your burn. This can be done a few times each day until the burn gets better.

- You may also take a lukewarm bath with a couple cups of apple cider vinegar into the tub to heal your burn. You can take two baths per day until your burn gets better.

As you can see, there are many different ways to use apple cider vinegar for beauty reasons.

Chapter 4: Natural Cures with Apple Cider Vinegar

Apple cider vinegar, as you should know by now, is a highly versatile liquid and can be used for your health, cleaning, and as food. Natural health enthusiasts everywhere celebrate the healing abilities of apple cider vinegar for nearly every problem.

This chapter will cover how you can use apple cider vinegar to detox and cleanse your body.

The Miraculous Cleansing Abilities of ACV:

Using apple cider vinegar can help you clean your body because of its content of enzymes, vitamins, and minerals. It will detox your body, removing toxic waste and getting rid of bacteria before it can cause a lot of bodily damage to you.

Apple cider vinegar both improves bowel movement and aids digestion, detoxifying your liver, improving your body's circulation, and purifying your blood. It has strong enzymes that help to break down harmful cholesterol and keep it from clogging up your body and arteries.

How else does it Help your Body Detox?

Apple cider vinegar helps to maintain a positive alkaline pH balance to keep away inflammation in your body. Inflammation is caused by high levels of acid.

Apple cider vinegar also helps to clean your lymph nodes and break up the mucus present in your body, which then improves your immune system and lymph circulation. We've already covered the ways that apple cider vinegar can aid you with weight loss.

It allows your body to more effectively break fast down, rather than storing them on your body. It's also full of pectin to keep you fuller for longer, reducing water retention and suppressing an overactive appetite. If you combine apple cider vinegar with the right nutrition and exercise, it can help tremendously with keeping the fat away.

As mentioned before, selecting the right kind of this vinegar is a must for achieving the results you dream of. True apple cider vinegar is created by a fermentation process that turns apples into vinegar.

Simple Apple Cider Recipes Anyone can do:

Never choose pasteurized vinegar or the type that comes in a plastic bottle. Each time you use your organic apple cider vinegar, don't forget that you should shake the glass every time in order to get as many good elements as you can.

Using apple cider vinegar Internally:

Apple cider vinegar is highly acidic, so make sure you dilute it with water before drinking so your esophagus and teeth stay safe. Even though apple cider vinegar is acidic, it does create an alkaline effect in your body when ingested.

The fact that this liquid has an alkalizing impact on your body has a large effect on its abilities to heal so many ailments.

Don't Use too much:

You should never use too much of this liquid, just dilute a couple of tablespoons in a big glass with water, drinking it before or during meals twice per day.

Ingesting apple cider vinegar in typical food amounts is mostly very safe, as long as you don't use too much. Drinking too much of this daily could lead to health issues like a lower bone density or lowered levels of potassium.

In addition, apple cider vinegar can cause interactions with some medications, so ask your doctor before taking it with heart meds or diuretics.

An Eternal Apple Cider Vinegar Bath:

The skin is your biggest organ and has a lot to do with how effectively your body can detox. Although not everybody enjoys steam rooms or can access them, you may begin to cleanse your body at home in the tub.

True, not everyone likes the smell of apple cider vinegar, but its benefits are so plentiful that it's worth it. If you're very bothered by the scent, just add some essential oils to your bath. You may also add some herbs.

- Just add the raw apple cider vinegar to your tub, then let it soak in there for a minimum of 15 minutes. This is highly effective for fighting skin irritation and bacterial infections because of its antimicrobial benefits.

- This bath can be taken two times per week to help balance your skin's pH level and cause softer, nicer skin.

<u>Making your Own Apple Cider Vinegar Detox Beverages:</u>

Not everyone can stand the taste of apple cider vinegar diluted with just water, so if you're one of these people, you will surely appreciate the following recipes.

An Apple Cider Vinegar and Lemon Drink:

Lemon water is another liquid that helps immensely with weight management, digestion, and other health issues. This beverage has some cinnamon in it, too, which metabolizes glucose in your body to help prevent the storage of fat.

Cinnamon also aids your digestion to help you feel full and stay that way for much longer. The drink has cayenne pepper for bringing your body temperature up, which makes your body work to get it cool again.

During this process, the body must burn a higher number of calories as it cools down, helping you shed some extra weight.

The Ingredients Needed:

To make this drink, use a glass of filtered water, one tablespoon of lemon juice, one tablespoon of organic, high-quality apple cider vinegar, half a teaspoon of cinnamon grounds and a pinch of cayenne.

You may also add stevia, quality maple syrup, or another natural sweetener. Don't use typical sugar. This should be stirred together and drank immediately.

Your Detoxing Cranberry Beverage:

Water and raw, healthy cranberry juice can help you clean out your kidneys, bowels, liver, and your lymphatic system of harmful, bad toxins.

Cranberries are full of compounds that draw fat out of your lymphatic system, since one of your lymphatic system's functions is absorbing fats from your digestion system, bringing them to your blood circulation.

For the cranberry juice you use, ensure that it's unsweetened, organic, and pure. Here are the ingredients for you detox beverage:

- One tablespoon of lemon juice.

- One tablespoon of apple cider vinegar.

- Half a cup of organic cranberry juice.

- Some water.

Mix the ingredients with as much water as you want until it tastes the way you prefer. You may make it strong or weak and flavor it with pure honey.

Your Weight Loss Green Tea Beverage:

Green tea helps you burn fat by boosting the metabolism. The mixture of honey, apple cider vinegar, and green tea combine to create a weight management drink that will also help you suppress your appetite.

Keep in mind that mixtures such as this work much better when combined with healthy eating habits and plenty of exercises. Before adding the apple cider vinegar to your tea, ensure that it's cooled enough and is no longer boiling, or it will ruin the apple cider vinegar's active culture.

Here are the ingredients you need to create this wonderful beverage:

- One tablespoon of apple cider vinegar.

- A single cup of organic green tea.

- Honey, if you prefer.

Make a cup of green tea, add some honey, then allow the tea to cool down. Add the apple cider vinegar to the mix. You can drink this right away to receive the benefits.

Vinegar Drizzle to cure your Sore Throat and Aid Digestion:

If you have issues like acid reflux (which can happen from not having enough acid in the stomach), ulcers, or colitis, apple cider vinegar mixed with some fermented vegetables can ease many different stomach issues.

The gentle acid present in fermentation is known as lactic acid, not acetic acid and can help to balance and heal the gut microbiome. Studies done on animals have shown that apple cider vinegar helps with digestion.

One study showed that apple cider vinegar could help ulcerative colitis by helping overall digestion issues. The study discovered that adding acetic acid to water helped bring better bacteria levels to the mice's guts.

In order to help your overall gut health, just make a concoction that consists of two tablespoons of apple cider vinegar, a glass of warm water, and a small amount of organic, raw honey.

Apple cider vinegar with ginger and honey for throat soreness is also effective and highly popular. You can also use this mix to help your sore throat, which comes recommended by a nurse from Pittsburgh University, Bonnie K. McMillen.

- Two tablespoons of pure water.

- One tablespoon of apple cider vinegar.

- A quarter teaspoon of powdered ginger.

- One tablespoon of organic, raw honey.

- A quarter teaspoon of cayenne pepper (optional).

To get the best results from this recipe, just take small sips once every two or three hours, swallowing it very slowly, so it has plenty of contact with your sore throat. Instead of directly sipping apple cider vinegar, dilute it with water.

A Vegetable Drizzle:

A yummy and simple recipe to put over salad greens, asparagus, or broccoli is a tablespoon of lemon juice, a tablespoon of apple cider vinegar, half a tablespoon of fresh, minced garlic, a bit of basil, and some black pepper.

If, after using apple cider vinegar for a while, you still don't like the taste, there are a few other creative ways you can ingest the liquid. Let's look at them now.

A delicious Cranberry Cocktail:

To make this tasty beverage, just mix together the following ingredients:

- Two tablespoons of organic cranberry juice.

- Half a cup of water.

- Two tablespoons of apple cider vinegar.

- Two tablespoons of organic maple syrup.

Mix all of these ingredients together in a glass and drink it immediately. Cranberries are a great addition since they are full of antioxidants, help heart health, aid digestion, and help to heal urinary tract infections.

Sweet, Mineral-rich Blaster Beverage:

This drink is not only sweet and tasty, but it's highly effective to help clean your body out. Here are the ingredients you will need to make it:

- Two tablespoons of molasses (black strap).

- Two tablespoons of apple cider vinegar.

- Two cups of water.

Blend these ingredients together and drink them right away. For the best results, you should take this first thing in the morning after waking up. It will deliver the great health advantages of apple cider vinegar while also bringing your body more calcium, manganese, magnesium, and iron from the molasses.

A Tomato Juice Lover's Drink:

This one won't be the favorite taste of most apple cider vinegar drinkers, but if you enjoy tomato juice, you will probably like it very much. Here are the ingredients you need to make it:

- Two teaspoons of fresh sea salt.

- Two tablespoons of organic apple cider vinegar.

- Canned or fresh tomato juice (as much as you want).

- Some hot sauce (if you prefer that).

This can be mixed together and drank immediately between meals.

Super Tangy Pink Juice:

To make the next item on our list, just gather and combine the following substances:

- Two tablespoons of organic, raw honey.

- Two tablespoons of apple cider vinegar.

- 1.5 cups of organic, fresh grapefruit (pink).

Blend all of this together in a glass and drink it down. You can use this before each meal during the day. If you want to lose some weight, this is very helpful. In addition, grapefruit can help you lower cholesterol while preventing arthritis and some forms of cancer.

A Simple Apple Cider Vinegar Shot:

For those who prefer a simpler method instead of an elaborate concoction, this shot may be perfect. Just mix together these ingredients to get the benefits of apple cider vinegar directly:

- A single tablespoon of apple juice or water.

- One tablespoon of organic apple cider vinegar.

Blend these two together and drink it back right away. You can hold your breath or plug your nose if you don't like the taste.

Increase the Brightness of your Chili:

Next time you're cooking chili at home, you can use apple cider vinegar as a way to increase flavor and brightness.

Apple cider vinegar can not only be used as a mouth rinse or whitener but may be used to clean your dentures or toothbrush. Just soak the brush in half a cup of water with a couple tablespoons of apple cider vinegar, then a tablespoon of pure baking soda.

Again, keep in mind that this acidity may cause tooth erosion, as proved in a single study. Another way to use apple cider vinegar is to kill your weeds, particularly the pesky ones growing on your sidewalk or driveway. Weed killers full of chemicals may harm your water system.

<u>Natural Cures with Apple Cider Vinegar:</u>

Apple cider vinegar is useful for may different conditions and can also be used as a strong cure and alternative to sometimes harmful traditional medical treatments.

As mentioned, you may use it to clean your house, your toothbrush, to kill weeds, and more! In addition, health professionals use it to target ailments and enhance changes in your lifestyle. Odds are, the liquid may enhance at least one area of your life. Here is a list of ways to use apple cider vinegar.

- **A Possible Remedy for Hair Loss:** We mentioned earlier that apple cider vinegar could help your hair become shinier and cure dandruff, but did you know that it can also be used as a remedy for hair loss?

  Simply add some apple cider vinegar to your hair, diluted with water, after you give it a regular shampoo and enjoy these benefits! Make sure you rinse well to get the smell out or use essential oils to make it less harsh.

- **A Strep Throat Remedy;** Most of us have had this common issue at least once in our life, but the powers of apple cider vinegar are very effective for treating it.

  Just mix some apple cider vinegar with warm water in a glass and gargle it a few times per day. How much you need depends on whether you're used to the liquid, but between one and three tablespoons should be sufficient.

- **Aiding Sinus Issues and Infections:** Traditionally, apple cider vinegar has been used to help treat sinus infections. To help your sinus infection disappear, just dilute a few tablespoons of apple cider vinegar in a glass of warm water.

You may also mix some organic honey into it to make the taste nicer. This could cause your infection to be healed within just three days or so.

- **Healing Congestion Issues:** Apple cider vinegar has plenty of potassium, as we've mentioned, and this nutrient can help your body's mucus production decrease over time.

  In addition, apple cider vinegar has acetic acid that can help kill the growth of bacteria, including the bacteria responsible for nasal congestion issues. Drink some a couple times each day right before going to sleep diluted in water and mixed with organic honey.

- **Minimize your Pores:** In order to keep your pores looking nicer and smaller, just dab apple cider vinegar onto your face, diluted in water. You may also mix some baking soda in. Be sure to follow up with a quality, natural moisturizer.

- **Minimize Stretch Marks:** In order to make your stretch marks fade, just mix some apple cider vinegar with two parts warm water, blended with some raw honey. Put this in your stretch marks, leaving it to sit for two minutes before rinsing it off.

  Don't expect this to completely diminish your stretch marks, but it can help a lot with making them less noticeable.

- **Foot Fungus:** Along with curing foot odor, apple cider vinegar can help heal athlete's foot and other foot fungus problems. Just let your feet soak in a mix of warm water and vinegar, but don't pat dry after. Instead, let it dry on its own.

- **Curing the Hiccups:** One study showed that a teenager with a chronic hiccup issue solved the problem by mixing sugar and apple cider vinegar. Hiccups are the result of eating too much food, digesting sugary, fatty foods, or a low level of acid in the stomach.

  You can use apple cider vinegar to cure these, since it restores your stomach's balance of acid, easing the diaphragm spasms, and also triggering mouth and throat nerves, which contribute to the hiccups.

- **Helping Ear Infections:** As mentioned before, apple cider vinegar is a quality disinfectant. You may mix together water and rubbing alcohol, putting it into your ears with a dropper. Many people use this as a home remedy since it acts very fast compared to other methods.

- **Curing the Cold:** Apple cider vinegar works to boost your immune system, both protecting and strengthening your body when you get the cold or a flu.

Of course, many other home remedies with apple cider vinegar exist than just these ones, but it's a good start! It's a great remedy to use at home since it's cheap, easy to make, and very natural.

Here are some other Ailments that ACV can Help with:

- Menstrual cramps.

- Diabetes problems.

- A cough.

- Cleaning your wounds.

- Soothing mosquito bites.

- Bee stings.

- General inflammation and itching.

- Body detox.

Recommended Apple Cider Vinegar Brands

Apple cider vinegar on a regular basis can help you feel healthier and more energetic. You will be able to more effectively digest your food, feeling way lighter after eating.

You must also do conscious exercise and eating choices to get the full benefits. For years now, people have been reporting their amazing results from using this common, natural health remedy.

For many centuries, this vinegar has been put to use as a magical health tonic, curing high cholesterol, weak immune systems, heart issues, skin problems, diabetes, high blood pressure, and much more.

It can also be used to make your skin more youthful, to help combat hair loss, and to help you lose weight. Studies show that drinking this liquid each day can help you keep your blood sugar under control.

<u>More Purported Apple Cider Vinegar Benefits:</u>

- Treating varicose veins.

- Lowering blood pressure issues.

- Reducing cholesterol.

- Keeping osteoporosis away.

- Curing Psoriasis.

- Removing muscle stiffness.

- Soothing tired muscles.

- Strengthening your teeth and bones.

- Anti-aging effects on the skin.

- Helping to nourish your plants.

- Making your hair shinier and longer.

- Building up your immunity.

__The Right Apple Cider Vinegar to Purchase:__

Apple cider vinegar shouldn't be confused for white vinegar, which is found in the majority of home kitchens. Although, as mentioned before, all vinegar is pretty healthy, white vinegar is more useful for cooking, washing, and cleaning the house.

However, this vinegar has usually been refined, and therefore, doesn't have as many health advantages as pure, organic apple cider vinegar.

More about Apple Cider Vinegar:

Apple cider vinegar is made from a mix of crushed apple parts, also called apple must. This results from crushing entire apply, along with the seeds, stem, and skin.

The apple is brought through fermentation and oxygenation, converting the apple sugar into alcohol first. As it oxygenates, the present alcohol is changed into acetic acid, leading to the health values we've been discussing in this book.

Of course, the value is only retained when the vinegar is made the right way and is sold with the mother. So what is important to search for when purchasing apple cider vinegar?

Buy Organic:

Although this isn't an absolute must, it's best to buy your apple cider vinegar from organic apples, which will have natural sugar and no pesticides. In addition, the businesses that utilize organic apples probably take the care to follow a quality process for creating their apple cider vinegar.

Buy Unfiltered:

Buying unfiltered apple cider vinegar will help you make sure that it has the mother still in it, which is the muddy, grainy substance at the bottle's bottom. When you shake this up, the mother will float. The mother is the foundational essence of all apple cider vinegar, which stores the enzymes and provides all of the benefits you desire.

Buy Unpasteurized:

Always buy apple cider vinegar that is not pasteurized. The pasteurization process heats the liquid and kills of bad forms of bacteria, but unfortunately, this also gets rid of the bacteria you want.

Since you now know to search for unpasteurized, unfiltered, and organic apple cider vinegar, what brands should you look for? When it comes to choosing the right brand, keep in mind that more expensive doesn't always mean better. Actually, more affordable brands often give better value for what you pay.

The Best Apple Cider Vinegar Brands:

Here are some of the best apple cider vinegar which also offer you affordability:

Bragg Apple Cider Vinegar:

Bragg is among the absolute oldest of apple cider vinegar brands available today. Bragg is also very trusted in terms of vinegar brands. The company is based in California and uses apples that are native to the U.S.A. Due to this, they can control the quality of the apples they use.

Only organic apples are used, meaning that they don't have any pesticides or arsenic in them. In addition, Bragg uses wooden barrels to boost the fermentation process.

Bragg was founded by a man named Paul C. Bragg who advised some Olympian athletes, and his brand is backed up by his nutritionist daughter, Patricia Bragg.

Vitacost Apple Cider Vinegar:

Although Bragg is well-known for its range of apple cider vinegar, the brand Vitacost sells other health products, in addition, with the vinegar only being one purchase choice. Actually, Vitacost is more preferred than Dynamic Health and Bragg apple cider vinegar brands.

Vitacost says that the apple cider vinegar they make is the result of fermenting freshly pressed apples that are completely organic. The apple cider vinegar is not pasteurized, meaning it still has the mother. It has no sugar added, no colors added, and no artificial flavorings. In addition, it's suitable for vegetarians along with being kosher. For those seeking a quality, cheap brand, Vitacost is a great option.

Fleischmann's Apple Cider Vinegar:

You may also purchase apple cider vinegar from Fleischman's. This brand is based in California and has been creating vinegar since back in the 1920s. The brand started out using alcohol from the growth of baker's yeast.

As technology has advanced, baker's yeast lowered the alcohol production, causing the brand to enter into the specialty of creating just vinegar.

Dynamic Health and Apple Cider Vinegar:

Dynamic Health was created in 1994 and has been providing products and health supplements that are halal-certified, fully organic, and also available in both capsule and liquid forms.

The apple cider vinegar products from Dynamic Health are very competitive, offering quality value for what you spend.

To Summarize:

To summarize, each of these brands covered are great. The companies use organic, fresh-pressed apples that create unpasteurized, unfiltered, raw, organic apple cider vinegar. Each of these still has the healthful mother intact.

You don't have to store your purchased apple cider vinegar in the fridge, but you should avoid sunlight and keep it in glass rather than plastic.

<u>Where to Buy Apple Cider Vinegar:</u>

Apple cider vinegar can be made on your own, as we covered earlier in the book, but you can usually find it at health food stores, online, or even at ordinary grocery stores. In order to find a quality brand, you will probably have a better look at a specialty health store.

Chapter 5: Precautions and Recommendations

Apple cider vinegar not only has amazing health benefits but is completely safe to ingest. However, if you aren't careful, some side effects could occur. Do the side effects from apple cider vinegar mean that it isn't safe to ingest? Let's look at the details of this question.

Let's first be clear on one thing; apple cider vinegar is very safe to ingest. A wonderful supplement for great health, the benefits of apple cider vinegar are very numerous.

From utilizing it to tone your skin to making your hair nicer, and also to help you lose weight, you shouldn't miss out on apple cider vinegar. So why is there some concern about how safe consuming apple cider vinegar is, along with possible side effects?

There's a simple answer to that question. Apple cider vinegar is acidic, so consider the following before committing to a daily supplement of it.

<u>What Amount is Safe to Consume?</u>

Consuming too much apple cider vinegar can hinder your body from effectively and fully absorbing calcium. For this reason, don't take over 30 ml per day.

When should it be Ingested?

As stated and shown, apple cider vinegar has many benefits, but it's best to consult a doctor if you have any concerns or questions about whether it's right for you.

This is especially important if you want to use it to cure stomach ailments, kidney problems, wart removal, liver detox, sore throat problems, or to control your blood sugar.

When shouldn't you use ACV?

Although drinking apple cider vinegar in a safe, recommended amount, in some cases, there isn't a lot of information freely available on how safe it is to consume apple cider vinegar.

If a woman is breastfeeding or pregnant, she shouldn't consume too much apple cider vinegar unless her doctor specifically suggests or approves it. In addition, if you have a disease of any kind, please consult your doctor before you ingest this liquid to prevent any side effects from occurring.

Now that you are aware of some of the side effects that may come from apple cider vinegar, you should know more about it before drinking it regularly.

Some of the Possible Side Effects of Apple Cider Vinegar:

Low Levels of Potassium:

Since apple cider vinegar is so acidic, one common issue with ingesting too much of it is lowered levels of potassium in your blood. If you have been drinking apple cider vinegar and notice low blood pressure, cramps, or nausea, please ask your doctor to look into the reasons behind this. It may be due to consuming too much apple cider vinegar.

Irritation of the Throat:

As mentioned earlier in the book, apple cider vinegar can bring relief to throat soreness, but consuming it too much could lead to the opposite effect, irritating your throat and worsening the condition.

Lowered Density in the Bones:

Excessive use or over-dosage of this liquid could lead to lowered bone density in your body. It could make your bones weaker, indirectly increasing the risk of breaking your bones from a hard fall or minor accident.

Erosion of Tooth Enamel:

We already briefly discussed the risk of your tooth enamel being eroded from too much apple cider vinegar. Even soda heightens the risk of tooth erosion because of the drink's acetic makeup.

In a similar way, apple cider vinegar being used often isn't very different and can lead to both decay and the general erosion of your teeth.

Causing Skin Irritation:

If you use apple cider vinegar for your skin, particularly on the sensitive skin of your face, be careful. If you have sensitive skin, it's best to first consult an expert. As said before, always dilute this liquid before you apply it to your face reducing the risk of skin burn or irritation.

<u>Taking Precautions before Use of ACV:</u>

- Make sure you avoid using ACV without dilution unless a health expert or doctor has specifically guided you to do so.

- Don't ever consume apple cider vinegar more than the safe, recommended amounts or it could cause your body harm.

- In order to gain the full possible health benefits of apple cider vinegar, it's best to ask your doctor how much he or she recommends that you take. This way, you will stay safe and reduce risks of health problems.

- Keep in mind that apple cider vinegar is very safe for your body as long as you follow these guidelines for safe consumption.

Once you observe all of the rules above, you should be fine to drink apple cider vinegar every day.

Chapter 6: Bonus: Apple Cider Vinegar in Treatment of Cellulite

Cellulite is an embarrassing problem that affects many people, mostly women. Cellulite consists of fat cells under the skin that are free floating. The appearance of cellulite is very distinct and appears like cottage cheese or a dimpled orange peel surface. Genetics, hormones, and a lack of healthy habits are the main causes of this problem.

You have to get rid of it right away when it shows up because cellulite usually worsens as you age. There are a few different effective methods that can pause or slow down this occurrence, minimizing the look of cellulite on your body, especially on the thighs.

Apple cider vinegar is one effective method for doing that. We will discuss how and then give some other natural remedies for curing cellulite. For the best results, use these in combination.

How does Apple Cider Vinegar helps with Cellulite?

Apple cider vinegar contains strong astringent properties, along with its previously mentioned skin-toning abilities that will help your body get rid of cellulite, the freely floating cells of fat just below your skin.

There are several components present in apple cider vinegar that can help water retention and with flushing out toxins near your stomach and thighs, which goes a long way to reducing the unattractive look of cellulite. Along with this, apple cider vinegar aids in weight loss, improving your skin's elasticity.

<u>Your Home Cellulite-Busting ACV Recipe:</u>

In order to reap the benefits from this wonderful liquid to fight your cellulite, just follow these very simple instructions:

- Mix three parts apple cider vinegar with one-part coconut or olive oil, then place this in the area that is affected.

- Massage the mixture into your skin for 15 to 20 minutes. This can be repeated two times per day until you see an improvement.

- You may also mix two tablespoons of unfiltered, raw apple cider vinegar with a teaspoon of organic, raw honey in a warm glass of filtered water. This can be drunk twice per day, every day.

This drink will help your body fight imbalances in your hormones, which can lead to a weight gain issue.

<u>How Does ACV Help Remove Cellulite?</u>

Apple cider vinegar helps your body get rid of this problem because of the calcium, magnesium, and potassium present within it. Each of these elements contributes to flushing toxins out of your body, along with reducing water retention in both the stomach and the thighs.

This process helps to reduce cellulite and general body bloating, helping you shed extra pounds. Lower amounts of fat on the body means lower pockets of cellulite on the body.

Here is a useful recipe for helping to reduce cellulite, which can be used in conjunction with the one above:

- Combine two parts warm water with one-part ACV. You can optionally add raw honey, too.

- Spread this mixture over your affected body areas and allow it to sit for a half hour. It can then be rinsed off using lukewarm water.

- Do this twice a day to reach your desired result.

- On the other hand, you can mix water with apple cider vinegar in two equal amounts, rubbing it over your thighs or other areas of cellulite.

- This body part should be wrapped up in Saran wrap, then rinsed off with water. This can be done once per day until your cellulite goes away.

Note that you may also add a teaspoon of raw honey to two tablespoons of ACV, drinking this twice a day, every day.

Other Natural Remedies for Cellulite to use with ACV:

Apple cider vinegar isn't the only useful ingredient for helping you fight cellulite. You may use the following remedies to make the apple cider vinegar treatment even more effective.

Using Coffee Grounds to Fight Cellulite:

You can use coffee grounds to make an exfoliating body scrub. This will take away old, dead cells of the skin, generate healthier, newer cells. In addition, drinking coffee often can help improve your body's blood circulation. Just follow these steps to gain the wonderful cellulite-blasting properties from coffee:

- Combine olive oil or liquid coconut oil (two tablespoons) with three tablespoons of raw sugar and a quarter cup of coarse coffee grounds (fresh or used). Once this paste is blended, it can be spread over the affected area.

  Allow this to sit for a few minutes after you apply it with firm pressure, then rinse the mixture off your skin with warm (not hot) water.

- This solution can be used up to three times each week to get the results you desire. Keep in mind that you can store any leftover materials in a jar to use later.

- In addition, you may create an olive oil and coffee warp. Just heat up a bit of virgin olive oil with half a cup of coarse coffee grounds in your microwave. Don't heat them for over 20 seconds or it will get too hot.

- This mixture should be spread over your cellulite, then covered up with Saran wrap. Allow it to sit for a half hour before rinsing it from your body. This can be done twice weekly until your cellulite improves.

Using Juniper Oil to Heal Cellulite:

Juniper oil contains many valuable detoxifying ingredients, helping to fight fluid retention, which in turn can treat cellulite in your body. To make use of this amazing oil, just follow these steps:

- Combine 15 drops of this oil in a quarter cup of melted coconut oil or organic olive oil.
- Spread this oil over your cellulite and let it sit for 15 minutes each time you use the treatment.

- This can be done two times each day. Once 30 days have passed, your skin in that area will appear firmer and softer to the touch.

Using Seaweed to Fight Cellulite:

Seaweed is a useful and natural agent of exfoliation for the skin. It helps your body stimulate blood circulation, flushes out toxins, and improves the texture of your skin. All of this combines to help reduce the look of your cellulite. Just follow these steps to benefit from seaweed for fighting cellulite:

- Combine a few tablespoons of seaweed (make sure it's ground) with a quarter cup of extra virgin olive oil and a quarter cup of pure sea salt. This can be found in most health stores in America.
- You may mix some of your favorite essential oils into this mix to make it smell nice, then rub it onto your cellulite, leaving it to sit for 15 minutes and then rinsing it off in a warm shower.
- Once this has been applied and you have rinsed it off, make sure you use a moisturizer to heighten the effects.
- This natural remedy can be utilized every day for weeks at a time, and the extra mixture may be stored away in an airtight container to use later on.
- In addition, you may bathe with some seaweed in the water, which can help you reduce cellulite on your body. To do this just add a few sheets of seaweed into your tub, then fill it with warm or hot water.
- Soak in your tub for at least a half hour and perform this two times a day to get the highest number of benefits.

Cellulite can be a really embarrassing problem, leading you to want to hide your body and avoid swimsuits. You shouldn't have to live with this anymore, and with these natural recipes, you have a way to naturally change that.

Using some of these suggested natural remedies you now have the potential to remove cellulite within just a month: combined with a healthy diet, lifestyle and moderate exercise routine.

..And don't forget to use apple cider vinegar for all of the other amazing benefits we've covered throughout this book. Good luck!

<u>Conclusion</u>

Thank you for reading *Apple Cider Vinegar: Natural Weight Loss, Glowing Health and Skin, Natural Cures, and Alkaline Healing with Apple Cider Vinegar.*

<u>Taking Action For Your Health:</u>

Hopefully, this book has shown you some of the many ways that you can start to use the wonderful apple cider vinegar to improve your health and improve your life overall. Making this miracle liquid at home is very simple and easy, and that way, you can be sure it's organic and raw

Whether you want a chemical-free method for cleaning your kitchen, wish to help cure your acne, or want to lose some weight, apple cider vinegar can help!

Finally, if you found this book enlightening and useful, please take the time to leave a positive review on Amazon. Thank you and good luck!

www.ingramcontent.com/pod-product-compliance
Lightning Source LLC
Chambersburg PA
CBHW071212240726

48654CB00009B/747